PALLIATIVE CARE

This book is d···

CURRENT CLINICAL ONCOLOGY

Maurie Markman, MD, SERIES EDITOR

For other titles published in this series, go to
www.springer.com/series/7631

PALLIATIVE CARE

A CASE-BASED GUIDE

Edited by

JANE E. LOITMAN

*Department of Neurology, Washington University
School of Medicine, St. Louis, MO, USA*

CHRISTIAN T. SINCLAIR

Kansas City Hospice, Palliative Care, Kansas City, MO, USA

MICHAEL J. FISCH

*Department of General Oncology, The University of Texas
M.D. Anderson Cancer Center, Houston, TX, USA*

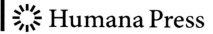 Humana Press

Editors
Jane E. Loitman, MD, MS, FAAHPM
Department of Neurology
Washington University
School of Medicine St. Louis, MO, USA
loitmanj@gmail.com

Christian T. Sinclair, MD, FAAHPM
Kansas City Hospice
Palliative Care
Kansas City, MO, USA
csinclair@kchospice.org

Michael J. Fisch, MD, MPH, FACP
Department of General Oncology
The University of Texas
M.D. Anderson Cancer Center
Houston, TX, USA
mfisch@mdanderson.org

ISBN 978-1-60761-589-7   e-ISBN 978-1-60761-590-3
DOI 10.1007/978-1-60761-590-3
Springer New York Dordrecht Heidelberg London

Library of Congress Control Number: 2010927098

Printed on acid-free paper

Humana Press is a part of Springer Science+Business Media (www.springer.com)

Preface

A clinical case-based handbook has a role in general clinicians' practice of caring for patients with serious or life-limiting illness. The explosion of the field of Hospice and Palliative Medicine impacts all physicians and healthcare providers. Fellowship trained specialists graduate in greater numbers annually. These and more seasoned specialists are now certified by the American Board of Medical Specialties as subspecialists. Research in this field is expanding in scope and quantity, and peer reviewed journals devoted to this work are multiplying. Moreover, peer reviewed journals in primary care and other subspecialties of medicine regularly include papers that focus on end-of-life care, quality of life issues, and symptom management. Overall then, access to clinical information necessary to care for patients with life-limiting illness is not only essential, but also increasingly available.

This case-based clinical book aims to help with the actual practice of caring for patients with life-limiting illness. Numerous texts and journals exist to provide the data to inform care, yet there remains a need to find practical points and information about the practical application of the principles of palliative care. Thus, we hope that the cases, key points, and practical tips will help health care providers who are not experts already in palliative care in the care of patients with serious illness and challenging problems. Some chapters follow one patient through the course of an illness to highlight the applicability of palliative care throughout the disease process. Whether with one patient or with several patient examples, clinical aspects are highlighted.

Some aspects of Hospice and Palliative Medicine remain in transition or relate to individual practice style. To put the data and other more global topics into perspective, the nature of these issues is addressed. Similarly, the less recipe-driven areas of care such as communication, the terminal state, and bereavement are included to provide a framework to approach these situations.

Physicians and other healthcare providers crave data. Each section includes a brief list of papers or chapters from textbooks providing more substantive data. Hopefully, this handbook will help you provide care in the patient's room, home, or exam room and then provide further tools for exploration once back to your library, office, or computer.

St. Louis, MO   *Jane E. Loitman*
Kansas City, MO   *Christian T. Sinclair*
Houston, TX   *Michael J. Fisch*

Contents

Contributors

CLAY M. ANDERSON, MD • *Division of Hematology and Medical Oncology, Missouri Palliative Care Program and Department of Internal Medicine, Ellis Fischel Cancer Center, University of Missouri, Columbia, MO, USA*

MILES J. BELGRADE, MD • *Pain and Palliative Care Center, Fairview Health Services, Minneapolis, MN, USA*

GARY BUCKHOLZ, MD • *The Institute for Palliative Medicine at San Diego Hospice, San Diego, CA, USA*

TERESA DESHIELDS, PhD • *Psycho-Oncology Service, Alvin J. Siteman Cancer Center, St. Louis, MO, USA*

MICHAEL J. FISCH, MD, MPH, FACP • *Department of General Oncology, The University of Texas M.D. Anderson Cancer Center, Houston, TX, USA*

JOSHUA HAUSER, MD • *Department of Medicine, Buehler Center on Aging, Health and Society, Palliative Care and Home Hospice Program, Northwestern University, Feinberg School of Medicine, Chicago, IL, USA*

JANE E. LOITMAN, MD, MS, FAAHPM • *Department of Neurology, Washington University School of Medicine, St. Louis, MO, USA*

KARIN B. PORTER-WILLIAMSON, MD • *Department of Internal Medicine, University of Kansas Medical Center, Kansas City, KS, USA*

ERIC ROELAND, MD • *Department of Hematology and Oncology, University of California San Diego, San Diego, CA, USA*

DREW A. ROSIELLE, MD • *Department of Medicine, Palliative Care Center, Medical College of Wisconsin, Milwaukee, WI, USA*

CHRISTIAN T. SINCLAIR, MD, FAAHPM • *Kansas City Hospice and Palliative Care, Kansas City, MO, USA*

MARISSA SLAVEN, MD • *Division of Palliative Care, Department of Family Medicine, McMaster University, Hamilton, ON, Canada*

DAVID WENSEL, DO • *Hospice & Palliative Care, Mercy Medical Center – North Iowa, Mason City, IA, USA*

CYNTHIA A. WORLEY, BSN, RN, CWOCN • *Division of Nursing, The University of Texas M.D. Anderson Cancer Center, Houston, TX, USA*

1 Global Palliative Care Issues

Marissa Slaven

ABSTRACT

Palliative care for a patient is provided by an interdisciplinary team of health care professionals whose composition and roles may vary but whose goal is to provide whole person care. Traditional research and evidence-based practice is an exciting but very new development in palliative care. Therefore, research into the best practice in palliative care faces many unique challenges. Grief is a normal response to loss that involves processes and tasks at emotional, cognitive, and behavioral levels. The initial shock of learning of impending or actual loss necessitates creating a new relationship between the grieving person and the person (or object) of loss. Patient and family grieving processes can be aided by a wide variety of healthcare and community services.

Key Words: Care provider; Palliative care; Bereavement; Loss; Grieving; Healthcare; Community services; Whole person care

> *Mr. J is a 69-year-old father of four with a 4 month history of newly diagnosed, metastatic cholangiocarcinoma. He has not had and is not eligible for any disease modifying treatments and is being cared for at home. He is able to acknowledge his terminal illness and he wishes to be kept comfortable.*

CONSIDER

1. What is the evidence base for the palliative treatments offered?
2. What role do different care providers play?
3. What is the bereavement process and support before and after death?

From: *Current Clinical Oncology: Palliative Care: A Case-based Guide,*
Edited by: J.E. Loitman et al. DOI: 10.1007/978-1-60761-590-3_1,
© Springer Science+Business Media, LLC 2010

KEY POINTS

- Grief is a normal response to loss which involves processes and tasks at emotional, cognitive, and behavioral levels. The initial shock of learning of impending or actual loss evolves into a process of creating a new relationship between the grieving person and the person (or object) of loss.
- Patient and family grieving processes can be aided by a wide variety of healthcare and community services.
- Palliative care is provided by an interdisciplinary team of health care professionals whose composition and roles may vary but whose goal is to provide whole person care.
- Traditional research and evidence-based practice is an exciting but very new development in palliative care.
- Research into best practice in palliative care faces many unique challenges.

SCENARIO 1:
EVIDENCE-BASED PALLIATIVE CARE TREATMENT

Mr. J reports significant abdominal pain, bloating, and constipation. He has knife-like intermittent pain in the right upper quadrant and constant aching lower abdominal pain which he rates as 8/10. He gets some relief with hydromorphone 2 mg every 4 h as needed and is on long acting hydromorphone 6 mg twice daily. His last bowel movement was more than 7 days ago. He takes 3 senna tabs three times a day as well as lactulose 15–30 cc twice per day. He has no nausea or vomiting but his appetite is poor. X-rays of his abdomen show a moderate amount of stool.

Historically, studies of medications and interventions in palliative care are infrequent and tend to have small numbers of patients. Until the recent past, palliative care was not associated with mainstream or academic medicine. There were few scientists or clinicians with knowledge of both research methodologies and palliative care. There was little or no funding publicly or privately to support research in this new field. Additionally, there was a significant concern about the ethics of conducting research in this patient population. Consequently, most palliative care interventions have been based on level C or D quality data (small non-randomized studies or best expert opinion). With the growth of the field in the last decade, more specific and actionable research questions are being asked and institutions are growing to sufficient size to enable high quality research.

You suspect Mr. J's constipation is contributing to his pain, bloating, and poor appetite. The patient's opioids are likely a contributing factor to the constipation. You suggest methylnaltrexone, a newly approved medication for treating opioid-induced constipation.

Prior to gaining FDA and Canadian Health Protection Board approval for use in opioid-induced constipation, methylnaltrexone was studied in a double-blind, randomized, placebo controlled phase III trial at 27 US and Canadian nursing homes, hospice sites, and palliative care centers. It is the progression to this level of research which will enhance the ability of palliative care providers to ensure the best possible care for patients and families.

Clinicians and researchers are beginning to perform more diverse studies, including randomized clinical trials, as hospice and palliative medicine has grown and matured as a medical subspecialty with the development of fellowship training programs, American Board of Medical Specialties board certification, professional associations, and journals. Additionally, in the past 8 years reports from the Institute of Medicine, the Research Task Force of the American Academy of Hospice and Palliative Medicine, and the NIH have identified the critical need for palliative research and have called for major investments in palliative medicine research. A recent review of such funding revealed 75% of published palliative care research from 2003 to 2005 was funded, with one third of this funding coming from the NIH.

The complexities of ethical issues particular to palliative care research are well documented. Two of our preeminent colleagues offer a brief comment and response:

> To research the needs and experiences of this client group could be said to affront the dignity of those people who are terminally ill and an expression of profound disrespect for the emotional and physical state of such patients…one wonders whether they (research questions) should ever be asked by the living of the dying.
>
> (E Cassell 1991)

> We disagree with this distinction. The terminally ill are living. Furthermore, the suggestion that others have the right to deprive them of making their own decisions regarding whether they wish to participate in clinical research is paternalistic, demeaning and disrespectful. The frailty of the very ill does not preclude autonomous decision making, participating in society, giving to others or finding purpose and meaning.
>
> (Mount 1995)

SCENARIO 2:
INTERDISCIPLINARY TEAM CARE

Mr. J and his family have agreed for end-of-life care to be provided at home by his family, his family physician, and the palliative care-hospice team. After the team helped Mrs. J become familiar and comfortable with providing his nightly care needs, she is able to sleep for the first time in months. Certainly, without this much needed rest and support Mrs. J would not have been able to continue to attend to her husband's needs.

As Mr. J becomes more ill, he is unable to eat and was taking only small sips of water. The patient's Rabbi calls the palliative care physician to discuss issues of nutrition and hydration at the end of life. They are in agreement and are able to provide theological and medical explanations to help soothe the distressed family.

Mr. J dies peacefully in his own bed with his wife and four grown children at his bedside.

The team is a group of individuals working together with a common purpose. In this example, we see patients and families surrounded by an interdisciplinary health care team as well as members of their own community who worked together to allow patients to die comfortably in their own home.

Interdisciplinary team members	
Patient and family	Chaplain
Physician	Volunteer
Nurse	Physiotherapist
Social worker	Occupational therapist
Dietician	Pharmacist

Cassell suggests profound illness is associated with losses affecting all aspects of a patient's life. Significant losses are likely to injure the patient's entire sense of personhood – the complex interrelated physical, social, emotional, and spiritual dimensions which make up each person. Because palliative care focuses not just on relieving physical pain but on alleviating the suffering experienced by terminally ill patients and their families, effective interventions require the skills and resources of an entire team of healthcare professionals. Each patient and their family are evaluated separately by at least the core members of the team. Ideally, all members of the interdisciplinary team communicate well with one another to develop an interdisciplinary care plan. The care plan is negotiated with the patient/family to improve understanding and clarify roles and expectations. The care plan is often revised on a regular basis as the patient and family's needs change. Although time consuming, the multifaceted interventions are more likely to alleviate the factors contributing to patients' suffering.

The family is the most critical piece of the team providing care for the patient whether it is physical, emotional, or social. They will most often be the ones implementing the care plan proposed by the team. The interdisciplinary team needs to work with, educate, and support the patient's family as they too are experiencing stress, grief, and loss.

In the USA, the interdisciplinary team approach to caring for dying patients was institutionalized with the Hospice Medicare benefit in 1982. Reimbursement is tied to a hospice program's ability to provide an interdisciplinary team including the following core members: physician, registered nurse, social worker and pastoral, or other counselor as well as volunteers. For non-hospice palliative care programs, the composition of the team will vary depending on the stage of development of the program, the objectives of the program, and the needs of a given patient.

SCENARIO 3:
GRIEF

Mr. J's children approach the team nurse soon after the initial encounter. They express a mixture of concern and frustration with their mother, Mrs. J. She has remarked on multiple occasions she cannot imagine living without her husband of 46 years. They are concerned about suicide risk and frustrated because they felt their mother was at risk of taking attention away from the patient. The patient himself is concerned about his wife's inability to express acceptance of the prognosis. He also requested the team help his wife.

Grief is a normal response to loss, any loss: a job, a limb, a life. Clinicians have an important role in facilitating healthy grieving and observing for signs of complicated grief. Grief experienced by dying patients and loved-ones prior to death is called anticipatory grief and grief of loved-ones following a death is termed bereavement, which is usually accompanied by mourning.

Physicians can facilitate healthy grieving by being honest when discussing prognosis, goals, and treatment options; in fact, ambiguity from the physician may inhibit normal anticipatory grief.

When a patient expresses anticipatory grief, it can be confused with pain or depression. Grief tends to be experienced as sadness, whereas depression is associated with lack of self-worth. The question, "Are you sad or are you feeling depressed," may help begin a dialog to help you distinguish between grief and clinical depression.

(For more information on depression, see Chap. 4.)

The prebereavement period has been an important area of scientific investigations. A systematic review of research on the relationship between widowhood and emotional health found the relative risk of developing a mood or anxiety disorder was 3.5 to 9.8 times higher among recently widowed compared with nonwidowed. Married persons are at risk for spousal loss and may exhibit psychological and physical distress in anticipation of such an event. Research on marital transitions and health indicates married individuals have an increased prevalence of depressive symptoms preceding loss of a spouse.

Multiple members of the interdisciplinary team can be helpful to the patient's wife in her anticipatory grief including physicians, nurses, social work, and spiritual leaders. Communication amongst the members of the interdisciplinary team can facilitate this goal.

SCENARIO 4:
BEREAVEMENT

> *As Mrs. J gained trust in the team, she was able to discuss her inability to accept the patient's prognosis. She acknowledged his rapid physical decline and simultaneously expressed her sense of disbelief at the reality of the situation. She remained unable to envision her life after his death and until the last few days of his life was unable to truthfully tell him she would be alright after he died. She was unwilling to lie to him about this matter. When the patient died all of his family were present. The Jewish tradition of Shiva, sitting in mourning for 7 days, was observed giving family and friends' time to be together, to care for each other physically as well as emotionally.*

Bereavement and palliative literature suggests several different nonordered phases of grief. These include: numbness and blunting (sense of unreality), pining and yearning (emotional turmoil, crying, anxiety, anger), disorganization and despair (disengagement), and finally reorganization and recovery. Despite this "model" a great variation exists between people who may also move between phases.

To help people through this difficult transition formal bereavement support may be offered to loved ones by religious or community groups. Families of patients who had been enrolled in hospice can anticipate some bereavement support from the hospice program. Bereavement resources are also available through the Internet, and may fill a gap for family who are not able to access local or timely support. Funeral homes are another resource for families – both for direct support (through meetings and materials) and for referrals to other resources in the community. Another intervention which has been documented to aid in bereavement is dignity therapy, a process through which a legacy document is created with the palliative patient for the bereaved.

Bereavement occurs at a time when physicians and nurses who have supported families while the patient was alive are no longer involved in care. Intervention and support during this critical time can provide an opportunity to prevent ill health and to help people find new directions which may lead to psychological, social, and spiritual growth.

FURTHER READING

Appelbaum PS, Grisso T (1998) Assessing patients' capacities to consent to treatment. N Engl J Med 319(25):1635–1688

Cassell EJ (1982) The nature of suffering and the goals of medicine. N Eng J Med 306:639–645

Cassell EJ. The nature of suffering and the goals of medicine. Oxford: Oxford University Press, 1991, 27

Chentsova-Dutton Y, Shucter S, Hutchin S, Strause L, Burns K, Dunn L, Miller M, Zisook S (2002) Depression and grief reactions in hospice caregivers: from pre-death to 1 year afterwards. J Affect Disord 69(1):53–60

de Raeve L (1994) Ethical issues in palliative care research. Palliat Med 8(4):298–305

Health Care Finance Administration, Department of Health and Human Services. U.S. Code of Federal Regulations, Part 418 – Hospice Care. http://www.hospicepatients.org/law.html

MacDonald N, Hanks G, Doyle D (1998) Oxford textbook of palliative medicine, 2nd edn. Oxford University Press, New York, pp 103–107

Mount BM, Cohen R, MacDonald N, Bruera E, Dudgeon E (1995) Ethical issues in palliative care research revisited. Palliat Med 9(2):165–170

2   Palliative Care Communication Issues

Joshua Hauser

ABSTRACT

Difficult conversations for patients and families can be challenging for physicians and other healthcare providers as well. Optimal preparation for conversations about bad news, prognosis, goals of care, and hospice can make them more effective and less of a burden. The SPIKES strategy can assist in preparing and implementing these difficult conversations with patients and families. Effective communication can be made a priority by addressing issues proactively with colleagues.

Key Words: Goals of care; Conversation; Prognosis; Hospice; SPIKES strategy; Communication

> *Ms. A is a previously healthy 50-year-old schoolteacher who initially presented a seizure. A CT scan showed an enhancing mass and she was referred to a neurosurgeon for a biopsy.*

CONSIDER

1. How should a clinician prepare to break bad news to patients and families?
2. How does one help patients or families determine the goals of care?
3. What are some ways colleagues communicate with each other about patients near the end of life?

From: *Current Clinical Oncology: Palliative Care: A Case-based Guide,*
Edited by: J.E. Loitman et al. DOI: 10.1007/978-1-60761-590-3_2,
© Springer Science+Business Media, LLC 2010

2. KEY POINTS

- Difficult conversations for patients and families can be challenging for physicians and other healthcare providers as well.
- Optimal preparation for conversations about bad news, prognosis, goals of care, and hospice can make them more effective and less burden.
- The *SPIKES* strategy can assist in preparing and implementing conversations with patients and families.
- When getting a test with potential bad news, make a follow-up appointment to discuss the results so the patient does not need to wait for a phone call.
- Avoid superficially reassuring phrases such as "don't worry."
- Have certain phrases in mind before beginning this conversation; do not use these as a script, but consider them preparation.

SCENARIO 1:
BREAKING BAD NEWS

Ms. A's biopsy showed a high-grade glioblastoma multiforme and she has now returned for follow-up.

While it may be seen as a prototype for the act of "breaking bad news," a new malignancy is not the only type of bad news. Episodes of potentially difficult news include: the first discovery of a diagnosis, subsequent test results, changes in physical or cognitive condition, a transition of care from home to a nursing home, the lack of availability of further disease-modifying treatments, and the transition to hospice care. A strategy to deliver difficult news such as these examples is a skill commonly underdeveloped and therefore a situation often avoided by physicians and other health care professionals. This may be because of lack of comfort, lack of time, or lack of competence. Recognizing its importance and having a framework has been shown to help overcome these barriers.

SPIKES six-step protocol

1. Setting
2. Perception
3. Invitation
4. Knowledge
5. Empathy
6. Summary

One paradigm, developed by Robert Buckman, for breaking bad news is the "*SPIKES*" strategy. There are six steps in the preparation, discussion, and conclusion. In this framework, *Setting* describes the physical and temporal context in which one is delivering the news. *Perception* characterizes the patient's current understanding of the medical condition, treatment options, and prognosis. Perception can be addressed with an open-ended question such as "What have others told you about what is going on?" *Invitation* empowers the patient to define the amount of detail she prefers; for example, "Are you the kind of person who prefers to know all the facts about your illness or a more general description?" "How much information would you like me to give you about your diagnosis and treatment?" "Who else in your family is important for me to talk with?" *Knowledge* covers the aspect of communicating the difficult information. Most commentators suggest some kind of "warning shot" about news that is about to come: "Unfortunately, I've got some bad news to tell you, Mr. James." "Mrs. Haskin, I'm sorry to have to tell you...." After this introduction, the diagnosis or other piece of news should be delivered clearly, plainly and with a pause at the end of delivery. *Empathy* is the act of trying to connect with a patient on an emotional level, it may be mistaken for reassurance, but it is a much harder act since it involves understanding the patient without presuming to know exactly how she feels, "How does that make you feel?" "I imagine this must be difficult..." While empathy is considered the fifth step in Buckman's sequence, it is clearly an important bearing at each communication step. Finally, *Summary* refers to making clear follow-up plans regarding goals, treatments, and accessing resources.

SCENARIO 2:
GOALS OF CARE

Ms. A's glioblastoma was treated with surgical resection and a course of radiation therapy. She went home and comes in for a routine follow-up visit. She would like to return to work as a teacher and get back to normal. You realize the value of discussing the goals of care while she is feeling well, but are not sure how to start.

The idea of patients having dichotomous goals of cure at one point and comfort at another is outdated. In reality, most patients balance a mixture of these two goals throughout their illness. There is diversity in patient's goals of care and these goals are dynamic in nature depending on new medical results, social context, and evolving patient preferences. Therefore, it is never too early to discuss goals of care.

One of the foundational elements of palliative care is that aggressive life-prolonging and aggressive comfort treatments can occur concurrently. Patients may want both concurrently in order to achieve a specific personal goal, such as reaching a certain event or spending more time with a spouse. All members of the interdisciplinary team should strive to elicit patient's goals, understand and clarify them and advise patients about how to achieve them. One challenge is that the concept of "goals" may seem overly abstract. Therefore, when inquiring about goals of care, consider more concrete questions such as:

– "What is most important for you at this point in your care? What about if things should change?"
– "Are there specific things you want to do or accomplish?"

When asking this, physicians should both acknowledge uncertainty and help patients to think about the future. While "getting rid of the tumor" and "being cured" may be commonly hoped for treatment goals, you may need to insert the possibility of this not occurring. Even in the setting of a partial remission of a tumor, this can be done by using a phrase such as "I hope a cure might be possible, but I also want to help you think about if that doesn't happen...." You may also want to suggest more specific goals: being at home, going on a certain trip, seeing certain friends or family, finishing a specific project....

"From our talks before and from my sense of you from your daughter, it seems like something important to you at this stage is...."

Other pointers for these discussions include:

– Having ready examples of potential goals of care.
– Beginning with more open-ended questions, and following up with move specific questions.
– Acknowledging uncertainty and changing goals.
– Asking for specific goals and tasks.

SCENARIO 3:
DISCUSSING HOSPICE

Several months later, Ms. A has become increasingly tired and has lost 20 pounds. She subsequently has a seizure and is admitted to the hospital. A head CT shows tumor recurrence. Her oncologist believes her current performance status makes her a poor candidate for further disease-modifying therapy. You agree that her prognosis is less than 6 months. You visit her in the hospital to discuss next steps.

For many patients and families, hospice may be seen as another piece of bad news. As such, it is important to go back through the *SPIKES* protocol. As part of this, a crucial element is prior experiences with hospice for themselves, family members, or friends. For some, hospice is associated with giving up and abandonment; for others, it may be associated with emotional and practical support. These associations may not be an abstraction. Since more than 1/3 of deaths are currently cared for by a hospice at some point in their course, increasing numbers of patients and families will have experience with hospice and hearing about their experience is vital for physicians. A patient with a relative who died comfortably and peacefully with hospice care will have a very different association with the idea than one who felt abandoned and "left to die" because her doctors did not know what to do.

In the *SPIKES* framework, this is part of the *Perception* step. This can be done simply and straight-forwardly: for example, "A lot of people have had experiences with hospice. Have you? What were they like?" You may even want to be more specific and ask something like, "Were there things about hospice that were particularly helpful? What were they? Were there things about hospice you found less helpful? What were they?" These phrases both allow you to connect with the patient and also get a concrete sense of experiences and expectations of hospice.

Before even introducing hospice, however, establishing a context is important: this includes review of the goals of care, the medical facts, including the lack of available disease-modifying treatments or the recommendation that further treatment for the cancer is likely to be ineffective. The goals of care may help to integrate prior conversations with a change in treatment goals. "I know we've discussed what's important for you. I think hospice may be one way to achieve these things." Know general outlines of the services that hospice can provide and be prepared to discuss how you will integrate and coordinate with the hospice team.

SCENARIO 4:
PROGNOSIS

> *At the end of your conversation about hospice, Ms. A asks, "How long do you think I have to live?" How do you answer her?*

For more than a decade, there have been data to suggest that not only are physicians poor at formulating a prognosis, but they are also poor at discussing prognosis. Patients want our accuracy, our candor, and an acknowledgment of uncertainty. A phrase such as "I have no idea, I'm not God," is not a helpful one since it gives no overall idea of prognosis and actually underplays the amount we do know. At the other extreme, a phrase such as "2 months" or "6 months" can be overly exact almost ensuring the inaccuracy of the statement. Presenting the percentages is also of limited value.

Some clinicians prefer using ranges of time that are based on populations of similar patients. There are various prognostic scales, such as the "Palliative Prognostic Index" for patients with cancer that can give overall estimates for populations of patients based on disease and performance status and comorbidities.

In conversations where a new diagnosis or a change in status is presented, patients may want to know prognosis but be afraid to bring it up: A helpful phrase is "Some patients want to know about their prognosis (or 'life expectancy'). Is that something that would be helpful to you?" By asking this, a physician can give the patient the option of not hearing about it. If the answer is yes, presenting your best estimation using ranges, such as hours to days, days to weeks, weeks to months, months to years, is most helpful. If the prognosis changes, make sure to review the updated prognosis and the underlying reasons for the change to help patients and families appreciate the dynamic quality of prognostication.

Aside from the exact information, the nature of the request is important. The question of prognosis can be motivated by issues that are financial, physical, emotional, legal, or existential. If a physician only presents numbers, then the real question may not be answered.

SCENARIO 5:
TEAM COMMUNICATION

> *Ms. A is being cared for at home with hospice. However, in the last several days, she has become increasingly agitated. Because of concern that this was due to increasing edema around her tumor, the dexamethasone was increased but the agitation continued. Haldol and lorazepam were both added with minimal improvement.*
>
> *After extensive discussion with her family, a decision was made to admit her to inpatient level of care with the treatment goal of tapering of her steroids and symptomatically treating her agitation, with an understanding that she might die during the admission. Her hospice nurse discussed this with the admitting physician. He signed out to the physician covering for the night that "there's a hospice patient who is coming in for agitation."*

> *That night, the covering physician found Ms. A to be agitated with right-sided hemiparesis and an expressive aphasia such that she could not effectively communicate. Given her known glioblastoma, an additional 20 mg of IV dexamethasone was given and the patient's condition began to improve such that she was more alert and less agitated.*
>
> *The next morning, her family appeared and said, "I thought that she was dying and now and now she's more alert. This wasn't what we wanted and wasn't what she would have wanted."*

What Happened and How Can We Communicate Better as a Team?

Clinician–patient communication is classically regarded as a core competency in medical care of every sort. Less attention is often paid to communication between team members. This communication must be efficient and thorough if complex care is to be delivered safely and effectively. In this case, communication went from hospice nurse to the inpatient physician. There was a dropped hand-off between the two physicians resulting in a medical error (giving dexamethasone) in the treatment that this patient received.

Specific clinicians may have preferred ways of communicating and different disciplines may have different styles. Nurses, for example, may prefer to sign-out or "hand-off" by voicemail or tape-recorder, while physicians may prefer to be paged. Some clinicians are most comfortable face-to-face, while others prefer email messages. When "hand-offs" do occur, it must be clear who the recipient is and the type of information is conveyed in a compatible style.

Physicians tend to hand-off medical data in bullet points. Nurses may convey more varied information in full sentence format. Rarely do physicians include the goals or intent of the treatment in sign-out unless it relates to future treatments. Developing clear protocols around team communication is vital because missed information, especially about patient preferences and goals of care, can change treatments as it did in this case. This may be especially true in end-of-life care as the treatment goals for symptom management are frequently not congruent with acute care, disease-modifying goals. Since goals may be less obvious and more nuanced, a communication tool that includes goals of care as well as more traditional treatments is vital. Also in the hospice and palliative care setting, there is interdisciplinary hand-off which highlights the need for efficient communication between providers. Therefore, it is helpful to have clear protocols for hand-offs that include both medical details and goals of care.

FURTHER READING

Buckman RA (2005) Breaking bad news: the S-P-I-K-E-S strategy. Commun Oncol 2:138–142

Casarett DJ, Quill TE (2007) "I'm not ready for hospice": strategies for timely and effective hospice discussions. Ann Intern Med 146:443–449

Kaldjian LC, Curtis AE, Shinkunas LA, Cannon KT (2009) Review article: goals of care toward the end of life: a structured literature review. Am J Hosp Palliat Care 25:501

Lamont EB, Nicholas A, Christakis NA (2003) Complexities in prognostication in advanced cancer, "To help them live their lives the way they want to". JAMA 290:98–104

Lynn J (2001) Serving patients who may die soon and their families: the role of hospice and other services. JAMA 285:925–932

Stone C, Tiernan E, Dooley B (2008) Prospective validation of the palliative prognostic index in patients with cancer. J Pain Symptom Manage 35(6):617–622

3 Nutritional Palliative Care Issues

Clay M. Anderson

ABSTRACT

Food and nutrition have social, spiritual, and cultural overlaying meanings beyond their importance to the biological integrity of human beings. The balance of benefit and burden with natural and artificial nutrition and hydration is complex and dynamic. Total parenteral nutrition (TPN) may be helpful if the GI tract is not working and the illness and/or the complication is reversible and there is a reasonable likelihood of significant recovery. Oral, gastrointestinal (GI), or intravenous (IV) intake can be a net harm to the actively dying person who is not always capable of taking in or utilizing nutrients and water. Medical nutrition and hydration should cease before net harm occurs, but defining the moment of net harm remains a challenge to healthcare providers. The goals of nutrition should be considered in a patient with poor functional status and prognosis. Artificial nutrition and hydration should only be used as a bridge to attain a functional or quality of life goal as defined by the patient with a life-limited diagnosis. Artificial nutrition and hydration are optional at the end of life and the burdens and benefits must be considered. The perspectives of various stakeholders regarding the role of food and water, nutrition and hydration at the end of life are important to consider. Issues surrounding artificial nutrition elicit strong emotional responses, making effective communication with the patient/family unit about food and nutrition and fluid essential.

Key Words: Gastroinstestinal; Intravenous intake; Medical nutrition; Parenternal nutrition; Artificial nutrition; Tolerability; Toxicity

Mr. J is a 77-year-old widowed gentleman from a rural town. He has moderate dementia and has remained at home with his homemaker daughter and farmer son-in-law and three grandchildren. He is otherwise fairly healthy and has had a long but seldom utilized relationship with a family practice physician in town. With his daughter's prompting, he

From: *Current Clinical Oncology: Palliative Care: A Case-based Guide,*
Edited by: J.E. Loitman et al. DOI: 10.1007/978-1-60761-590-3_3,
© Springer Science + Business Media, LLC 2010

completed a living will and durable power of attorney for health care when his dementia was very mild. He recently had a large stroke, and is very debilitated and minimally responsive. He is not eating and is receiving intravenous hydration.

CONSIDER

1. The goals of nutrition in a patient with poor functional status and prognosis.
2. The options, burdens, and benefits of artificial nutrition at the end of life.
3. The perspectives of various stakeholders regarding the role of food and water, nutrition and hydration at the end of life.

KEY POINTS

- Food and nutrition have social, spiritual, and cultural overlaying meanings beyond their importance to the biological integrity of human beings.
- Actively dying patients are not always capable of taking in and utilizing nutrients and water.
- The balance of benefit and burden with natural and artificial nutrition and hydration is complex and dynamic.
- Effective communication with the patient/family unit about food and nutrition and fluid is essential.
- Oral, gastrointestinal (GI), or intravenous (IV) intake can be a net harm to the dying person.

  Medical nutrition and hydration should cease before net harm occurs.
  Defining the moment of net harm remains a challenge to healthcare providers.

- A natural and comfort-based approach in dying persons to food and water may require acceptance of the possibility of premature death.
- Artificial nutrition and hydration should only be used as a bridge in those with life-limiting diagnosis and should be associated with a functional or quality of life goal as defined by the patient.
- Issues surrounding artificial nutrition elicit strong emotional responses.
- Artificial nutrition and hydration generally are not helpful in dying persons.
- In dying patients, oral intake is usually preferred over NG tube, gastrostomy tube, IV administration based on tolerability, toxicity, risks, complications, and effectiveness.
- Total parenteral nutrition may be helpful if the GI tract is not working and the illness and/or the complication is reversible and there is a reasonable likelihood of significant recovery.

SCENARIO 1:
RELATED DEFINITIONS

After 3 days of minimal improvement and obvious clinical signs of aspiration, Mr. J and his family are approached by the primary team about a swallowing study and the possibility of a nasogastric (NG) tube and eventual percutaneous endoscopic gastrostomy (PEG) tube for nutrition. Mr. J is somewhat hungry and enjoying the food and fluids he is consuming, even with occasional coughing.

Anorexia is the lack of significant nutritional intake from any cause. Most anorexia is due to illness and disease which impairs appetite and digestion.

Anorexia nervosa is a psychiatric condition whereby a physically healthy, usually, young person severely restricts his or her oral intake of food to maintain a distorted body image.

Inanition is similar to anorexia but is the lack of oral intake of food or fluid.

Fasting implies volitional anorexia of any origin, usually of short duration.

Cachexia is a physiologic state in which loss of lean body mass and weight is due to the body metabolizing more calories than can be taken in. Initially, fat is lost, then muscle is broken down to provide energy, and the ill person loses weight, strength, and energy.

Early satiety is the sensation of fullness in the abdomen or stomach experienced before adequate nutrition in the form of food has been taken in by the oral route. Advanced disease, liver enlargement or upper abdominal masses, can cause the capacity of the stomach to diminish, thus not allowing the usual bulk of food to be taken in comfortably by the patient. In these cases, higher calorie and lower volume foods can be recommended. Also, smaller and more frequent meals can prevent or ameliorate weight loss or sometimes allow weight gain.

Artificial nutrition and hydration (ANH) is the medical application of caloric aqueous solutions or suspensions (nutrition) or noncaloric aqueous solution (water or saline or glucose solutions, serving as hydration) into the body through the gastric, intestinal, or intravenous route. This is in contrast to feeding the patient via the oral route with some form or normal or modified food and drink. When disease or the medical/surgical treatment of disease compromises the ability of the person to desire, take in, and use calories, protein, carbohydrates, fat, micronutrients, and water, it is sometimes necessary *to use AHN to support and rehabilitate the patient.*

SCENARIO 2:
HUNGER AND NUTRITION

Mr. J has a PEG tube placed and is fed with enteral nutrition around the clock. He improves modestly over a period of months. He is admitted with aspiration pneumonia 6 months later. He requires significant assistance with his ADLs and is incontinent of urine. His pneumonia responds well to antibiotics, but he is clearly declining. Hospice care is recommended as the best plan of care. His family agrees but they do not want to stop enteral nutrition. His daughter explains she does not want to prolong his life, but she feels stopping the "feeds" would be tantamount to murder since the nutrition is "keeping him alive." Without the "feeds" her concern is death and suffering by thirst and starvation.

Persons who are previously well and voluntarily refuse food and water can be expected to experience hunger and thirst. Similarly, persons who do not have access to food and water due to socioeconomic or personal circumstances will experience hunger and thirst.

Dying persons typically do not feel hunger or thirst when they refuse food and water due to poor appetite and lack of interest in food. Ad-lib oral intake, even when minimal, quenches thirst and satiates appetite in those with advanced illness. Typically, forcing oral, enteral, or parenteral nutrition into these persons does not satisfy cravings and tends to induce bloating, nausea, vague pain, and edema and compromises comfort. Forcing nutrition may also lead to seemingly unrelated conflicts between the patient and others secondary to the lack of control over their own body.

If recovery is the goal, food and water may still be indicated, but often comes at a cost of increased symptom burden. It is common for severely ill persons to not desire food and water and to not feel significant hunger or thirst if they take in only what they want or are able, including nothing for prolonged periods.

There are several barriers to usual oral intake of nutrition. Some persons may not have access to food and water. Others may have difficulties chewing or swallowing food or water for multiple reversible and irreversible reasons. In others, obstruction or dysfunction of the esophagus, stomach, or duodenum creates a barrier to oral nutritional intake. When the oral/enteral route cannot be used in a normal manner, it may still be used for pleasure, with caution and moderation. Much of the enjoyment of eating takes place in the mouth and is associated with texture and taste. When the gut does not work and the patient desires food, pleasure can be obtained orally but with the food then spit out. All barriers to oral intake should be overcome if possible without adding excess burden or undesired interventions.

If orotracheal or gastrotracheal aspiration is present as assessed clinically or radiographically, the patient is likely to develop aspiration pneumonitis or pneumonia, both without oral intake and much more so with oral intake. If this patient may recover or has goals of recovery/prolonged survival, then the oral route for nutrition and hydration must be enhanced (pureed or thickened food/liquid) or bypassed with NG or gastrostomy tube placement. The dying person will rarely be helped by such interventions, because they will not likely eat or drink much more anyway, will still aspirate even if without oral intake, and can often enjoy small amounts of oral intake without significant symptoms of aspiration. Antipyretics, pulmonary toilet, and occasionally antibiotics may help these patients avoid, or be comfortable despite, symptoms if they occur.

Patients, families, and nonmedical members of society in general spend much time planning for, preparing, and consuming food and beverage. Print, radio, and television media often focus on the same pleasures in life. Flourishing people eat well to live and live to eat and drink and be merry. We celebrate and grieve with food and beverage. Yet, pale colored, homogenous, thick liquid food (with or without fluids), delivered via tubing and syringes and bags and pumps, does not seem the same as food and in fact is a medical intervention just like *antibiotics or blood transfusions.*

SCENARIO 3:
CACHEXIA

Mrs. R is a 69-year-old woman who is dying of pancreatic cancer. She has always prided herself on her dress and style and has been active in church and in the community as a volunteer. Her pain and other symptoms are controlled. She is losing weight rapidly and her physical appearance is changing rapidly. This is frightening and upsetting to her. She has very little appetite. She eats until she is satisfied or feels full. She wishes she could gain weight and look normal again.

Questions

1. Can adding calories to her intake allow her to gain weight and improve her appearance?
2. What type of diet will help the most?
3. What about an appetite stimulant?

4. Does a feeding tube or TPN make sense?

5. How can we help her even if she continues to lose weight and muscle mass despite her and our best efforts?

6. In the normal state, the human body has homeostatic mechanisms to maintain fluid status and body habitus through thirst and thirst quenching, hunger, and satiety.

7. Internal physiologic cues are complemented by, and sometimes disrupted by, other internal and external cues that may alter drinking and eating behavior.

8. The external cues may be anything from smells, sights, and sounds, to television advertisements and snacks in the grocery checkout line, to stress from job or fear of bodily harm.

9. Cancer, heart failure, liver failure, kidney failure, severe dementia, and overwhelming infection (bacterial sepsis, influenza, malaria) are examples of disease states which cause the brain and body to change their signaling of need for sustenance and their ability to incorporate food and water into previously healthy body tissues.

10. Planned caloric increase with dietary teaching and oral supplements can restore this balance on occasion and allow weight stabilization and sometimes even some weight gain.

General Guidelines for Addressing Issues of Food, Water, Nutrition, and Hydration in the Terminally Ill

1. The best approach to nutrition and hydration in the person with life-limiting illness must be individualized.

2. Decisions made can always be reversed or superseded, and should usually not get in the way of initiating the best plan of care.

3. Talk about food and nutrition, water and hydration, and the important differences. Natural vs. artificial. Normal vs. medical. Clear language is very important.

4. Talk about the harms of undesired and unusable nutrition and hydration put into the body of an ill or dying person.

5. Talk about nutrition and hydration being used as a bridge to recovery. What type of recovery? Likelihood of recovery?

6. If ANH can help the patient achieve a realistic medical or personal goal, judicious use should be supported and prescribed, but not insisted upon.

7. If there is no real chance of survival or functional recovery, the bridge of nutrition and hydration is a bridge to nowhere, or worse, a bridge to more suffering and perhaps faster decline.

CONCLUSION

Mr. J and Mrs. R are living out a very important phase of their lives. They likely only have weeks to months of life left, so their time is precious. They deserve care and treatment that is in accordance with their wishes, effective, efficient, beneficial, safe, minimally burdensome, compassionate, and preserving and enhancing of their dignity. How natural food and water and ANH will be given and used by them is a critical aspect of their care. An underemphasized and understudied aspect of medical care, nutrition, and hydration principles and discussions can guide us to better care for our patients in an appropriate and patient-centered way if we take the time and effort needed.

FURTHER READING

Bryon E, de Casterle BD, Gastmans C (2008) Nurses' attitudes towards artificial food or fluid administration in patients with dementia and in terminally ill patients: a review of the literature. J Med Ethics 34:431–436

Casarret D, Kapo J, Caplan A (2005) Appropriate use of artificial nutrition and hydration – fundamental principles and recommendations. NEJM 353:2607–2612

Cochrane TI, Truog RD, Mareiniss DP, Glick SM, Casarett D, Kapo J, Caplan A (2006) Appropriate use of artificial nutrition and hydration. NEJM 354:1320–1321

Cravens D, Anderson CM (2003) Relieving non-pain suffering at the end-of-life. Mo Med 100(1):76–81

Hoffer LJ (2006) Tube feeding in advanced dementia: the metabolic perspective. BMJ 333:1214–1215

Mitchell SL (2007) A 93 year old man with advanced dementia and eating problems. JAMA 298:2527–2536

4 Psychiatric Palliative Care Issues

Jane E. Loitman and Teresa Deshields

ABSTRACT

Common psychiatric problems in cancer patients include depression, anxiety, sleep disturbance, and delirium. Yet the diagnosis of psychiatric disorders in the medical setting can be complicated by the symptoms of disease or the side effects of treatment. Somatic symptoms from cancer obfuscate the diagnosis of mood disorders and other psychiatric disorders. Valuable tools such as opioid analgesics, steroids, and anticholinergic medications may produce undesirable psychiatric side effects. Adverse effects (including delirium, mania, and depression) as well as milder effects (such as irritability, insomnia, and weight gain) may impair quality of life. One major challenge to psychiatric diagnosis presents itself during end-of-life care. In this case, it may be difficult to distinguish between primary psychiatric disorders and end-of-life distress. Psychosocial stressors, unrelated to disease or treatment, can occur and sometimes complicate management. Patients' reactions to recommended treatments may be related to other issues, such as grief, frustration, or need for control. As a result, the diagnosis of mood disorders may require input by mental health professionals.

Key Words: Treatment; Steroids; Mood disorders; Distress; Management; Psychiatric disorders; Side effects; Diagnosis; Somatic symptoms; Quality of life; Cancer

---

Mrs. JS is a 61-year-old woman previously diagnosed with lymphoma. Her disease has progressed and she has been advised to resume treatment. She has been married for 28 years and has three adult sons. She is attentive to her appearance and notes working as a model before she married. In the past, she was treated for Posttraumatic Stress Disorder related to a personal assault. During her previous treatment for lymphoma, she was prescribed steroids to reduce inflammation and nausea. She expresses concern about taking steroids again, knowing weight gain is a side effect.

From: *Current Clinical Oncology: Palliative Care: A Case-based Guide,*
Edited by: J.E. Loitman et al. DOI: 10.1007/978-1-60761-590-3_4,
© Springer Science+Business Media, LLC 2010

CONSIDER

1. The common iatrogenic psychiatric side effects of medications such as steroids
2. The distinctions between primary psychiatric disorders and end-of-life distress
3. The challenge of addressing altered mood in end-of-life care

KEY POINTS

- Common psychiatric problems in cancer patients include depression, anxiety, sleep disturbance, and delirium.
- Somatic symptoms from cancer obfuscate the diagnosis of mood disorders and other psychiatric disorders.
- Diagnosis of psychiatric disorders in the medical setting can be complicated by symptoms of disease or side effects of treatment.
- Valuable tools such as opioid analgesics, steroids, and anticholinergic medications may produce undesirable psychiatric side effects.
  - Addressing adverse effects may allow continuation of the causal agent, if required for symptom control.
- Patients' reactions to recommended treatments may be related to other issues, such as grief, frustration, or need for control.
- Steroids are commonly used in the treatment of cancer or other medical conditions, and for symptom management. Adverse effects, including delirium, mania, and depression, may impair quality of life.
  - Milder effects – such as irritability, insomnia, and weight gain – also impact quality of life.
- Emotional distress at the end of life is a symptom and should be treated as such.
  True mood disorders may require input by mental health professionals.
- Psychosocial stressors, unrelated to disease or treatment, occur and sometimes complicate management.

SCENARIO 1:
IATROGENIC PSYCHIATRIC SIDE EFFECTS

Mrs. JS completes the first 2 weeks of radiation treatment for her affected lymph nodes. She is taking steroids as prescribed. She comes in for routine follow-up. Her affect is sad, but she is fidgety and agitated. You complete a review of symptoms. She has gained weight. Upon questioning, she reports poor sleep with particular difficulty initiating sleep. Her interactions with you are curt and abbreviated. She fears being unable to complete radiation or chemotherapy and worries she will not survive her cancer.

The physical symptoms of disease or side effects of treatment can resemble signs of psychiatric disorders make assessment of psychiatric disorders complicated. Commonly used medications are frequently associated with neurocognitive side effects and therefore can mask early diagnosis of depression, anxiety, or delirium. Insomnia and increased appetite associated with steroid use may resemble the neurovegetative signs of depression (sleep disturbance, changes in appetite or weight, anergia). While most clinicians think of depression as characterized by psychomotor retardation, an agitated presentation is also possible.

Discontinuation of steroids may not be possible when they are used for disease modification; Symptom management, thus, becomes of prime importance. Additionally, agitation (and sometimes mania) induced by steroids disrupts relationships and is disconcerting for the family, caregivers, or health care providers.

Mrs. JS's initial concern about resuming treatment may reflect anxiety about a change in her prognosis with progression of her disease. Considering her longstanding attention to her appearance, sensitivity must be given to Mrs. JS's concerns about weight gain. In our current culture emphasizing informed consent, patients are typically given a lot of detailed and specific information. Many patients can be overwhelmed, and possibly discouraged by this. A brief discussion of both what type and how much information the patient would like to receive can make this type of communication with the patient more effective.

The clinician can be uncomfortable with patients' denial. Denial can be an effective protective mechanism that allows patients to process distressing information at a pace that they can psychologically handle. As long as the patient is keeping necessary medical appointments, there is no need to directly challenge the patient's denial. Alternatively, there is also no need to actively support denial by distorting test results or other medical information. Straightforward discussion, respecting the limits of how much the patient wants to know, can help patients come to terms with the reality of their situation at their own pace. (For more on communication, see Chap. 2.)

Medications can be used to help patients through acute, time-limited situations and medication-induced side effects.

- Benzodiazepines are effective for acute intervention with anxiety, agitation, or insomnia, although they may also cause agitation, delirium, or depression. For example, geriatric patients and those with any CNS pathology are most at risk for benzodiazepine-induced symptoms, considered as disinhibition of the frontal lobe's control over behavior or frontal-lobe release. Careful consideration of benzodiazepine use in these populations is warranted.
  - Lorazepam, in particular, is utilized most commonly in hospice and palliative medicine. Doses can start at 0.25 mg and be titrated to achieve the desired effect. In patients for whom a dose limit is desired secondary to concerns about overuse or adverse effects, orders can be written with a set maximum, for example, 0.5 mg every 2 h as needed, not to exceed 4 mg per day.
- Antidepressants can also be utilized to counteract agitation from steroids or other medications. SSRIs or SNRIs need higher doses for longer periods of time to positively impact anxiety or agitation. Trazodone, an older antidepressant, can also be utilized to calm patients at low doses, 25–100 mg every 6–8 h as needed.
- Antipsychotics such as haloperidol or olanzapine can also help with agitation, mania, delirium, or depression. Some antipsychotics carry black box warnings concerning increased risk of stroke in patients with dementia or other risk factors. In addition, nursing home regulations may complicate their use. Lastly, the stigma of a medication labeled as an antipsychotic can be a psychological obstacle for patients with a "medical illness."

Regardless of prescribing trends, each antipsychotic has specific advantages and disadvantages. Mrs. JS would benefit from an antipsychotic which is sedating but does not have significant weight gain or appetite stimulation side effects. Haloperidol, while older, would meet her needs. If she were further along in her illness and appetite stimulation were desired then olanzapine might be a better option. In palliative medicine, doses are usually much lower than that required for treatment of psychosis or schizophrenia. If well tolerated, doses can be titrated to achieve the desired effect or reduce the side effect(s) of concern.

SCENARIO 2:
ACUTE DEPRESSION

> *Mrs. JS's son was in a severe auto accident in another state. He is in critical condition, hospitalized in an intensive care unit and unlikely to recover. She missed a radiation treatment and comes to you, tearful, wanting to discontinue treatment to go to her son.*

It is important to note that the stressors of life can impact not only patient well-being but also compliance with and tolerance for treatment. Certainly, given Mrs. JS's history of PTSD, one is more concerned about severe reactions, such as suicidal ideation, to distressing events. Her safety must be assessed and assured, as suicide is not uncommon in palliative care patients.

Antidepressants can address the neurochemical components of depression and acute stressors but can take 2–6 weeks to achieve maximal dose effect. Doses may be increased or adjusted, but then require an additional 2–6 weeks latency to affirm efficacy. If more immediate effects are needed, a stimulant can be effective.

- Mirtazapine has more rapid onset of action than other antidepressants and may be considered first. The rapid effect may be secondary to improving sleep or appetite, or reducing nausea. At lower doses, mirtazapine has greater effects of sedation and appetite stimulation which may impart a sense of well being.
- Stimulants have been demonstrated to benefit cancer patients with fatigue and/or depression and have also been useful in other palliative settings. Methylphenidate can be started at 2.5 mg upon awakening and repeated in 4–5 h, with an almost immediate response. The dose can be titrated to maximize effect or minimize side effect.
- SSRIs or SNRIs can be chosen for their actual effects or to address side effects associated with a particular agent, although onset of action and both the frequency and quantity of the pill burden should be considered.
- Numerous adjuvants can enhance mood, such as lithium, thyroid supplementation, anticonvulsants, and neuroleptics. Specific medications should be chosen based on existing side effects and pill burden. Utilizing one adjuvant to address multiple symptoms (e.g., sleep and mood or pain and mood) is preferred.

For Mrs. JS, medication may not be sufficient to help her cope with her overwhelming circumstances; therefore, counseling is advised. A psychologist and/or licensed clinical social worker can help her sort out how to deal with the trauma in her family as well as how to cope with her diagnosis, changing roles, treatment burden, decision-making processes, and other psychosocial issues.

SCENARIO 3:
INSOMNIA AND DELIRIUM

> *Mrs. JS has completed radiation and 3 weeks of weekly chemotherapy. Her husband comes in to the oncology clinic and reports his wife has not been herself. She is awake during the night and saying "really odd things. In fact, last night she insisted she saw something that wasn't there."*

Sleep deprivation can produce a host of symptoms, including depression and cognitive dysfunction. Management of insomnia requires a thorough evaluation of psychological as well as medical symptoms. Sleep hygiene is important to review. The type of insomnia, whether initial insomnia, frequent awakenings or terminal insomnia, can help drive the treatment. For initial insomnia, a review of bedtime rituals and evening dietary intake may highlight a problematic agent such as caffeine or an interruption of the descent into sleep by stimulating activity such as watching television or reading something without convenient breaks. Similarly, anxious thoughts interfering with sleep may be addressed with cognitive restructuring. For frequent awakenings, patients should be directed to get out of bed if lying awake for 30 min and to engage in boring or sedating activities before attempting to return to sleep.

Pharmacologic selection should also be based on the type of insomnia.

- If cognitive-behavioral or sleep hygiene interventions do not resolve initial insomnia, then short-acting medications to induce sleep onset may suffice. Benzodiazepines are useful for acute or short-term problems. However, benzodiazepines disturb sleep architecture, which in turn affects the quality of sleep. Newer agents can help with sleep onset although cost may be an issue.
- For frequent awakenings, if cognitive-behavioral interventions do not suffice, choose a longer acting sedative. Older antidepressants, such as amitriptyline, nortriptyline, and trazodone, are effective alternatives, with a longer effect. Amitriptyline can be started as low as 5 or 10 mg (more typically 25 mg), nortriptyline at 10 mg, and trazodone at 25 mg. At these low doses, side effects which may be deterrents, to continued use, are lessened. Therefore, medication can be titrated to maximize effect or minimize side effect.

Delirium is marked by the presence of a new altered sensorium, which waxes and wanes. It can be challenging to differentiate delirium from severe sleep deprivation or from depression with psychotic features, both of which can also be accompanied by hallucinations or delusions. Depression tends to be associated with either insomnia or hypersomnia, but the presence of low mood can help to distinguish this from delirium. Regardless, psychotic or delirious features should be addressed and a neuroleptic is the most appropriate therapy.

- Haloperidol is the antipsychotic of choice according to NCCN guidelines and a Cochrane review. An antidepressant or an adjuvant can also be implemented if, after cognitive status improves, one is indicated.
- Since delirium is more common in patients with cerebral pathology, such as stroke, dementia, or metastatic disease, a thorough evaluation is warranted if consistent with the goals of care. Similarly, several studies have demonstrated a correlation between an episode of delirium and increased mortality, particularly in the elderly. A review of the goals of care and overall quality of life should be addressed if and when cognitive status resolves.

In a palliative setting, particularly at the end of life, steroids need not be discontinued if there is a positive effect and no adverse effects. If steroids are the likely cause of delirium, the risk/benefit ratio and goals of care should be reviewed.

SCENARIO 4:
TERMINAL DELIRIUM

Mrs. JS's disease continued to progress. She was admitted into hospice 6 weeks ago. She is now agitated and restless with an associated delirium. Mr. JS and their surviving sons call because her condition is disconcerting for them.

Antidepressants

	For depression *May require 2–6 weeks at a dose prior to antidepressant effect*	As adjuvants *May titrate as tolerated by patient to effect or side effect*	For anxiety *May require 12 weeks at a dose prior to anxiolysis, usually at higher doses*	For sleep *May titrate as tolerated by patient to effect or side effect*
SSRIs				
Paroxetine	20 mg PO QD, MDD 80 mg	20 mg PO QD, MDD 80 mg	20 mg PO QD, MDD 80 mg	
Escitalopram	10 mg PO QD, MDD 20 mg		10 mg PO QD, MDD 20 mg	
Citalopram	20 mg PO QD, MDD 60 mg	20 mg PO QD, MDD 60 mg	20 mg PO QD, MDD 60 mg	
Sertraline	50 mg PO QD, MDD 300 mg	50 mg PO QD, MDD 300 mg	50 mg PO QD, MDD 300 mg	
Other				
Mirtazepine	15 mg PO QHS, MDD 45 mg	7.5 mg PO QHS, MDD 45 mg	15 mg PO QHS, MDD 45 mg	7.5 mg PO QHS, MDD 45 mg
Trazodone			25 mg PO Q 8 h PRN, MDD 300 mg	25 mg PO Q 8 h PRN, MDD 300 mg
Venlafaxine	25 mg PO TID, MDD 375 mg		25 mg PO TID, MDD 375 mg	
Bupropion	150 mg PO QAM, MDD 450 mg		150 mg PO QAM, MDD 450 mg	
Duloxetine		30 mg PO QD, MDD 120 mg	30 mg PO QD, MDD 120 mg	
TCAs				
Amitriptyline		10–25 mg PO QHS (titrate q 3 D)		10–25 mg PO QHS (titrate q 3 D)
Nortripyline		10 mg PO QHS (titrate q 3 D)		10 mg PO QHS, (titrate q 3 D)
Doxepin		25 mg PO QHS (titrate q 3 D)		25 mg PO QHS, (titrate q 3 D)
Stimulants				
Methylphenidate	5 mg PO Q AM and titrate to effect/ side effect, dosing 1st dose upon awakening and a 2nd dose in 4 h	5 mg PO Q AM and titrate to effect/ side effect, dosing 1st dose upon awakening and a 2nd dose in 4 h		
Modafanil	200 mg PO QAM	200 mg PO QAM		
Adjuvants best utilized by psychiatrists				
Lithium				
Thyroid supplements				
Neuroleptics				
Anticonvulsants				

Terminal restlessness, terminal agitation, and delirium are similar terms to describe a cognitive and behavioral pattern commonly seen in people who are actively dying. As suggested previously, delirum is difficult to witness and families report delirium as one of the more stressful symptoms to observe in patients. In the active phase of dying, reversible causes of delirium are rare; therefore, the treatment is symptomatic. Staff should initiate environmental and pharmacologic interventions for the patient and provide education and support for loved ones and caregivers. (For more on the terminal state see Chap. 10.)

- Environmental interventions are focused on reducing stimulation for the patient. Provide a quiet room with low lighting and minimal traffic.
- Pharmacologic interventions include a neuroleptic, titrated to maximize effect. While haloperidol is the neuroleptic of choice, more sedation may be desired, particularly with an agitated delirium. Chlorpromazine, a sedating neuroleptic, can be useful in this setting. Alternatively, benzodiazepines may be added. Opioids or other symptom medications should be continued and titrated as indicated considering sedation may mask distress.

Psychiatrists can be critical adjunct team members for patients with advanced illness. When initial interventions are not effective, psychiatrists' facility with diagnosis and the nuances of psychotropic medications can be invaluable. Psychologists or counselors can provide great assistance with nonpharmacologic interventions for the patient as well as primary support for the patient's loved ones and caregivers. While personality disorders are not discussed here because they are uncommon, their presence in a medical setting or at the end of life creates many challenges. Mental health professionals should be consulted to assist in the care and management of these patients.

In the following charts, the typical starting dose as a new medication and the maximum daily dose (MDD) are listed. These lists are not exhaustive.

Benzodiazepines

Lorazepam	0.5 mg PO q4 h PRN, MDD 12 mg	Effect T ½ 3–4 h	Used for anxiety or sedation Alleviates anxiety associated with dyspnea, not the dyspnea itself
Diazepam	5 mg PO q 8–12 h PRN, MDD	Effect T ½ 6–12 h	Used for anxiety, sedation, muscles spasms, seizures
Clonazepam	0.5 mg PO BID	Effect T ½ 8–12 h	Used for anxiety, myoclonus, seizures Only available in pill form

Only the most commonly used benzodiazepines are listed though there are many.

Antipsychotics

Haldoperidol	0.5 mg PO,SQ, PR q4 h PRN, MDD 300 mg	Can dose 1–6 times per day Used for anxiety, delirium, psychosis, sedation, nausea, bowel cramping
Thorazine	12.5 mg PO, PR, SQ q 4 h PRN, MDD 800 mg	Typically dosed every 6 h Used for anxiety, delirium, psychosis, sedation, hiccups
Resperidone	0.5 mg PO QHS, MDD, MDD 16 mg	Typically dosed at bedtime or BID Used for delirium, psychosis, sleep Typically used at bedtime. Greatest risk of metabolic syndrome
Olanzepine	5 mg PO QHS, MDD 20 mg	Used for sleep, appetite stimulation, anxiety, psychosis, other adjuvant uses
Quietepine	25 mg PO QHS, MDD 800 mg	Typically dosed at bedtime or BID Used for sleep and psychosis. Lowest risk extrapyramidal SE

Sleep agents

Initial insomnia	Lorazepam Zolpidem 10 mg PO QHS PRN, MDD unknown Zaleplon 10 mg PO QHS PRN, MDD 20 mg Melatonin 8 mg PO QHS PRN, MDD unknown	See above
Frequent awakenings	TCAs	See above
	Trazodone	See above
	Mirtazepine	See above
Determine if pain is a component and address pain or other symptom		

Anticonvulsants

Pregablin	75 mg PO BID, MDD 300 mg	May titrate to effect/side effect
Gabapentin	100 mg PO TID, MDD 3,600 mg	Sedation limits compliance and quality of life
Topiramate	25 mg PO QHS, MDD 1,600 mg	May dose all at bedtime or in divided doses if tolerated/desired
Phenytoin	100 mg PO TID	MDD determined by blood levels and SE
Levetiracetam	500 mg PO QD, MDD 3,000 mg	May give TID
Carbamazepine	100 mg PO QD, 1,600 mg	Side effects limit use
Valproic acid	250 mg PO QD, MDD 1,000 mg	MDD may be determined by blood levels and SE

FURTHER READING

Block SD (2000) Assessing and managing depression in the terminally ill patient. Ann Intern Med 132:209–218

Casarett DJ, Inoye SK (2001) Diagnosis and management of delirium near the end of life. Annals Int Med 135(1):32–40

Emanuel EJ, Hauser J, Emanuel LL (2008) Palliative and end-of-life care: psychological symptoms and their management. In: Fauci AS, Braunwald E, Kasper DL et al (eds) Harrison's principles of internal medicine, 17th edn. McGraw-Hill, New York

McCusker J, Cole M, Abrahamowicz M, Primeau F, Belzile E (2002) Delirium predicts 12-month mortality. Arch Intern Med 162:457–463

Patten SB, Barbui C (2004) Drug-induced depression: a systematic review to inform clinical practice. Psychother Psychosom 73:207–215

Rousseau P (2000) Death denial. J Clin Oncol 18:3998–3999

5   Cardiac Palliative Care Issues

David Wensel and Drew A. Rosielle

ABSTRACT

Heart failure follows an unpredictable disease trajectory. Several models now exist to help with prognostication, but accurate prediction remains difficult. Symptom management for pain, dyspnea, and depression is the primary goal of palliative treatment. Palliative treatments for CHF can overlap greatly with disease-modifying therapies such as in the use of diuretics and vasodilators to improve edema and exertional dyspnea. Discussing goals of care along with advance care planning should be done before a crisis. Quality of life for patients should be discussed early in the disease trajectory of heart failure. Patient and family education about the terminal nature of heart failure, hospice as a treatment option, and deactivating implanted devices is critical.

Key Words: Heart failure; Symptom management; Diuretics; Vasodilators; Disease trajectory; CHF; Hospice; Dyspnea; Depression; Palliative treatment; Cardiac therapy

> *Mr. J is an 82-year-old male who is married with a history of congestive heart failure (CHF) and diabetes mellitus. He has an implantable cardioverter-defibrillator (ICD) device, inserted 5 years ago after he had sustained ventricular tachycardia during a hospitalization. He is admitted for dyspnea and fatigue with a 15 pound weight gain in the last 24 h. This is his fourth admission in the last 2 months for these symptoms.*

CONSIDER

1. The risks of mortality on hospital admissions
2. Symptom management in the face of maximum cardiac therapy
3. The patients' denial regarding mortality from CHF
4. At what point is hospice care appropriate

From: *Current Clinical Oncology: Palliative Care: A Case-based Guide,*
Edited by: J.E. Loitman et al. DOI: 10.1007/978-1-60761-590-3_5,
© Springer Science+Business Media, LLC 2010

KEY POINTS

- Heart failure follows an unpredictable disease trajectory.
- Several models now exist to help with prognostication but accurate prediction remains difficult.
- Symptom management for pain, dyspnea, and depression is the primary goal of palliative treatment.
- Device technology has improved survival for patients but has become a potential source of suffering as well.
- "Palliative" treatments for CHF overlap greatly with disease-modifying therapies such as in the use of diuretics and vasodilators to improve edema and exertional dyspnea.
- Patient and family education about the terminal nature of heart failure is critical.
- Discussing goals of care along with advance care planning should be done before a crisis.
- Quality of life for patients should be discussed early in the disease trajectory of heart failure.

SCENARIO 1:
ESCALATING SYMPTOMS IN HEART FAILURE

Mr. J is extremely fatigued and gets short of breath just sitting up. He has spent the last week at his home and the last 2 days at home in his recliner or bed. He has been unable to go anywhere due to his extreme fatigue. He has only been able to sleep 2–3 h at a time and awakens with pain and dyspnea. His pain is worse with movement of his legs, which are swollen. Mr. J's wife does not understand why this keeps happening to him. She reports that after he is admitted to the hospital, his symptoms only improve slightly. He reports that shortness of breath is his most troubling symptom for now. His wife reports that he does not interact with her as much and this is very distressing.

Foundations of palliative care in heart failure

- Assess for symptom burden
- Maximize effective treatments
- Provide prognostic information
- Discuss goals of care

Common symptoms of end-stage heart failure are pain, dyspnea, depression, insomnia, anxiety, anorexia, and fatigue. The range and magnitude of symptoms are similar to those found in patients with advanced cancer with or without heart failure. In addition, fluid retention is very common and leads to a multitude of distressing symptoms. These include lower extremity edema which is painful, can limit ambulation, and be complicated by painful venous stasis ulcerations. Fluid retention can also cause abdominal distention and ascites which worsen anorexia, nausea, and abdominal pain, and pulmonary edema causing cough and shortness of breath.

When assessing for symptoms in heart failure it is important to ask about physical function and limitations. Not only does this help establish overall symptom burden and targets for therapy (e.g., ability to walk to the bathroom without help), but it also provides an opportunity to assess family caregiver needs and safety issues in the home. Functional status also has important prognostic implications for patients with CHF. Patients may report a better functional status than his or her family, so include them in the conversation and ask about their perception of symptom burden and patients' care needs. The New York Heart Association (NYHA) classification system is a key tool in stratifying symptom severity in CHF, and focuses on restrictions in activity caused by heart failure symptoms such as exertional dyspnea and angina. Other useful tools to help clinicians assess and document functional status include the Activities of Daily Living Scale and the Palliative Performance Scale (PPS).

NYHA classification

- Class I: No limitation of physical activity
- Class II: Slight limitation of physical activity and symptoms with ordinary activity (e.g., climbing stairs)
- Class III: Marked limitation of physical activity and symptoms (e.g., dyspnea or angina) with ordinary activity (e.g., bathing, walking across room)
- Class IV: Inability to carry on any physical activity with discomfort and symptoms at rest

Activities of daily living scale

Criteria	4	3	2	1
Bathing	Independent	Uses a device	Needs personal assistance	Complete assistance
Dressing	Independent	Uses a device	Needs personal assistance	Complete assistance
Toileting	Independent	Uses a device	Needs personal assistance	Complete assistance
Transfer	Independent	Uses a device	Needs personal assistance	Complete assistance
Continence	Independent	Uses a device	Needs personal assistance	Complete assistance
Feeding	Independent	Uses a device	Needs personal assistance	Complete assistance

Palliative performance scale

%	Ambulation	Activity and evidence of disease	Self-care	Intake	Conscious level
100	Full	Normal activity NED	Full	Normal	Full
90	Full	Normal activity some evidence of disease	Full	Normal	Full
80	Full	Normal activity with effort evidence of disease	Full	Normal or reduced	Full
70	Reduced	Unable to do normal work	Full	Normal or reduced	Full
60	Reduced	Unable for most activities significant disease	Occasional assistance	Normal or reduced	Full
50	Mainly chair	Minimal activity extensive disease	Considerable assistance	Normal or reduced	Full +/− confusion
40	Mainly bed	As above	Mainly assisted	Normal or reduced	Full or drowsy +/− confusion
30	Bed bound	As above	Total care	Reduced	Full or drowsy +/− confusion

(continued)

(continued)

%	Ambulation	Activity and evidence of disease	Self-care	Intake	Conscious level
20	Moribund	As above	Total care	Sips	Full or drowsy +/− confusion
10	Moribund	As above	Total care	Mouth care only	Drowsy or coma
0	Death	0	0	0	0

Start in the upper left column and work right. Go down in each column to the qualifying state before moving right.

SCENARIO 2:
TREATING THE HEART FAILURE TO TREAT THE SYMPTOMS

> *As you talk with Mr. J and his wife, they begin to report the extreme burden his care has become to them. His wife starts to cry and reports that she cannot take care of him anymore. She is unable to lift him and admits that they have called the local fire department to help get him up after a recent fall. He has not been able to do any of his personal cares for at least a week now.*

The current evidence for symptom and mortality reduction in all classes of heart failure includes several classes of medications. Diuretics remain the primary treatment to reduce breathlessness, edema, and improve exercise tolerance. Loop diuretics are often first-line treatment. Thiazide diuretics can be given when patients become resistant to loop diuretics alone and the addition of potassium sparing diuretics can also increase diuresis.

There is good evidence that ACE inhibitors improve survival and symptoms in all classes of heart failure. Other vasodilating drugs such as hydralazine and nitrates can reduce cardiac after-load and can improve dyspnea and exercise tolerance in some patients. Beta-adrenergic blockers have now been shown to improve symptoms and reduce NYHA class along with mortality. Carvedilol is the only beta-adrenergic blocker that has been demonstrated to be safe and efficacious in NYHA class IV disease.

In select patients, device-based cardiac resynchronization therapy such as bi-ventricular pacing has been shown to improve symptoms and quality of life, but are best introduced before patients reach the final stages of illness. Angina from comorbid coronary artery disease or poor cardiac output also occurs in end-stage CHF. It should be treated with nitrates – similar to patients without end-stage illness – as well as with opioids for refractory symptoms.

SCENARIO 3:
PAIN AND DYSPNEA IN PATIENTS WITH CHF

> *Mr. J is having significant issues with pain interfering with sleep and quality of life. He has limited activity from his dyspnea so you discuss with Mr. J and his wife the possible use of an opioid for both his pain and dyspnea. They reluctantly agree to a trial of short-acting opioids. You also caution them about constipation and prescribe an aggressive bowel regimen.*

Pain is a very common symptom and under appreciated symptom described by end-stage heart failure patients. It can be caused by many factors including edema, peripheral neuropathy, debility, poor cardiac output, and cardiac angina. Acetaminophen is safe and well-tolerated, and is the first-line therapy for patients with mild to moderate pain. It should also be used as an adjunct to opioids for patients with moderate to severe pain, either as part of a combination pill (e.g., oxycodone 5 mg with acetaminophen 325 mg) or scheduled separately (e.g., 1,000 mg TID). Nonsteroidal anti-inflammatory drugs are contraindicated for all patients with advanced heart failure as they can precipitate renal failure and aggravate fluid retention.

Opioids are the treatment of choice for moderate to severe pain because of their efficacy, safety, and concomitant ability to decrease dyspnea. Opioids are likely underutilized due to reluctance of providers to prescribe them, and patient concerns about side effects and overestimation of the risk of abuse and addiction. These concerns should be preempted by careful counseling about the safety of opioids and generally manageable side-effect profile.

Distressing or limiting dyspnea that persists despite best efforts at optimizing a patient's heart failure medications should be treated with opioids. Small trials and extensive experience have shown that opioids are effective and well-tolerated in a variety of patients with advanced illnesses and dyspnea, including CHF.

Opioid dosing for both pain and dyspnea is the same in patients with CHF as with other illnesses. Increased caution is wise ("start lower and go slower") in patients with concomitant renal or liver failure. For opioid naïve patients, especially ones very concerned with side effects, doses as low as 2.5 mg of oral morphine can be initiated, at least to demonstrate tolerability.

SCENARIO 4:
WHEN CHF IS CONSIDERED IN THE TERMINAL PHASE

Mr. J has been on the maximum tolerated doses of diuretics, ACE inhibitors, and beta-blockers for the last 6 months with increases in diuretics at each admission. The addition of a thiazide diuretic has provided only modest benefit.

As the palliative care team works to support patients and their families, education about disease progression and prognosis is very important. Heart failure follows an unpredictable disease trajectory and is associated with a high incidence of sudden death. While many patients have a slow overall decline, punctuated by acute exacerbations with partial recovery, some patients remain steady for years and die in the setting of an acute decompensation. While all patients with a diagnosis of CHF should be counseled about its natural history including its life-limiting nature and the likelihood of sudden, life-threatening exacerbations, when to label someone as being in a "terminal phase" is more challenging. Nevertheless, the importance of addressing prognosis, goals of care, and treatment options becomes critical as a patient's overall condition worsens. Certainly, this discussion should occur with any patient whose functional status is not fully restored between exacerbations or who has a major, life-threatening complication from their CHF such as the need for ICU-level care.

Overall, patients with NYHA Class IV CHF have a 40–50% 1-year mortality (JAMA 04). Several models have been developed to help with short- and long-term mortality in advanced heart failure patients, but have not been validated in diverse patient populations. One study has demonstrated that the presence of at least three of the following factors was associated with a 40% 6 month mortality in older patients: renal failure, hyponatremia, systolic blood pressure <120 mmHg, and peripheral arterial disease.

Hospice care is appropriate for patients with a reasonable chance of dying within 6 months, and goals of care which emphasize quality of life and symptom relief over life-prolonging measures. Medicare provides criteria guidelines for admission to hospice with a diagnosis of heart disease provided if:

1. The patient has significant symptoms of recurrent congestive heart failure at rest and is classified as New York Heart Association (NYHA) Class IV. Assessment of NYHA class for prognostication reasons should be done when a patient is stable, and not in the midst of an acute exacerbation. Significant congestive heart failure may be documented by an ejection fraction of <20%, but is not required if not already available.
2. At the time of initial certification or recertification for hospice, the patient is or has been already optimally treated for heart disease or are patients who are either not candidates for surgical procedures or who decline those procedures. (Optimally treated means that patients who are not on vasodilators have a medical reason for refusing these drugs, e.g., hypotension or renal disease.)
3. Documentation of the following factors will support but is not required to establish eligibility for hospice care:
   • Treatment resistant symptomatic supraventricular or ventricular arrhythmias
   • History of cardiac arrest or rescuscitation
   • History of unexplained syncope
   • Brain embolism of cardiac origin
   • Concomitant HIV disease

Supporting evidence includes:

   • Frequent medication adjustments
   • Refractory edema
   • Dependent edema
   • Azotemia (elevated Blood Urea Nitrogen)
   • History of evidence of angina, arrhythmias, previous MIs

SCENARIO 5:
DISCUSSING PROGNOSIS AND CARE PLANNING

You begin the discussion about prognosis with Mr. J and his wife by asking them if they want to talk about it. They agree and when you ask Mr. J how he feels things are going, he immediately begins to cry. The palliative care team sits quietly as Mr. J begins to describe how poorly things have been going for him. He uses phrases like "quality of the time I have being more important than the quantity." He is very frustrated by not feeling better and wants to know why he can't seem to get stronger. When you inquire about what his understanding of heart failure is, he reports that no one has ever described it to him.

Many heart failure patients and their health-care providers do not think of the disease as a life-limiting, let alone terminal illness. When asked, patients with CHF report that it is important for them to know what their futures likely hold, including time-based prognoses.

Medical providers may discuss risks and benefits of individual treatments for CHF, but may not necessarily do so in the context of discussing a patient's overall prognosis and goals. Providers may also be reluctant to have these discussions due to the unpredictable nature of CHF, and concern for causing emotional harm to a patient. This can delay appropriate care planning and counseling about options, including refocusing of care toward symptom control, home safety, and support for family caregivers. Simply framing for a patient that his or her illness is incurable and life-limiting can be a powerful first step. Not all patients are ready to discuss these topics, but even bringing them up can communicate to them that you think they are worth addressing. Helpful initial questions can be: *Has anyone ever spoken with you about what to expect as your heart failure worsens? What worries you when you think about the future? Would you like to talk about what is likely to happen?*

Besides discussing prognosis, care planning for patients with advanced CHF should address:

- Eliciting patients values and preferences regarding balancing life-prolonging care with symptom relief in light of a poor prognosis
- Counseling about the benefits, burdens, and likely outcomes of the full spectrum of treatment options including ongoing efforts at life-prolonging care, care-focused solely on symptom relief without life prolongation, treatment limitations such as resuscitation orders and limiting rehospitalizations, and community-based care options such as home hospice and palliative care programs
- Counseling about completions of living wills, health-care powers of attorney forms, POLST documents
- Planning for crisis and encouraging patients to discuss with loved ones how they would prefer to be cared for in the setting of acute, life-threatening decompensations, especially if the physicians feel likelihood of recovery is small

SCENARIO 6:
DEACTIVATING DEVICES

Mr. J articulates that he feels he is dying and wants to focus his care on staying at home, getting as much help as possible to keep his symptoms under control, and getting help for his wife who is overwhelmed with his care needs. They are agreeable with hospice care, and he states he does not want to come back to the hospital, "As long as my wife can care for me at home." Mr. J says he does not want "any heroics" performed, and would like to die at home. You recommend, and he agrees with, a "do-not-resuscitate" order, however when you broach deactivating his ICD he appears surprised and fearful and indicated discomfort with such a plan.

The use of ICDs has expanded greatly in the last decade as the evidence supporting them as effective life-prolonging interventions in many patients with CHF has accumulated. Unfortunately, ICD firing is painful and frightening, and can cause anxiety and distress in many patients. In addition, patients may not understand fully the intention of ICD therapy, thinking instead that it is a form of "life-support" and that their heart will stop immediately without it. Patients and some providers can express ethical concerns of device deactivation as well, thinking that it is equivalent to "suicide" or "euthanasia."

There is broad consensus that similar to any other medical intervention, ICD therapy can be stopped in patients after an informed discussion with the patients or their decision maker about the potential risks and benefits of continued therapy. As patients die from any cause, the benefits of ICD firing (potential life-prolongation) become negligible, while the burdens (pain, anxiety, emotional trauma to loved ones) persist. Patients should be counseled about this, and given clear recommendations to stop ICD therapy when a clinician assesses the risk to be too great. Anticipate patient concerns that discontinuing ICD therapy will cause immediate death or is unethical, and counsel patients and families appropriately.

Pacing from an implanted pacemaker can also be ethically discontinued as it too constitutes a medical intervention any patient has the right to refuse after an informed discussion. In practice discontinuing pacing is less common, as it is not uncomfortable, and anecdotally many clinicians feel the symptom burden from bradycardia outweighs the benefits of stopping pacing in most patients. Most patients with pacemakers are not truly dependent on them for basic cardiac functioning, and it is unlikely that the dying process is substantially impacted by continuing or stopping pacing. Patients and families can be concerned that death will be needlessly prolonged by cardiac pacing, or may not understand how a patient's heart can stop beating even with ongoing electrical stimulation from the pacemaker. Careful about after counseling these issues is important, and deactivating a pacemaker is ethical and appropriate for patients who do not want to run the risk of any prolonging of death. In these circumstances, if the patient is felt likely to be symptomatic (as in the case of third degree heart block), it is important to have a plan in place for immediate symptom relief of dyspnea, dizziness, and angina.

In practice, discontinuing ICD or pacemaker therapy means deactivating the device via reprogramming it with a control device. Many patients have combination ICD-pacemakers, and the ICD function can be discontinued while keeping the pacemaker function active. Most patient's cardiology providers can do this in the clinic or hospital setting, and with adequate planning this can be done in the home setting as well. ICD technologists associated with device manufacturers can also do this, at times, with a physician's order. For patients who are dying with an active ICD who cannot have their device reprogrammed, placing a strong magnet over the implanted unit will deactivate the ICD function and any advanced pacing functions as well. This strategy can be helpful for patients dying unexpectedly in the hospital or home setting whose ICDs are firing and who do not have immediate access to reprogramming. Dying patients who are reluctant to have their ICDs deactivated for whatever reason, but who still wish to die at home, should be given magnets to keep in the home for emergency situations. Family caregivers should be instructed in how to use it.

FURTHER READING

Anderson F et al (1996) Palliative performance scale (PPS): a new tool. J Palliat Care 12(1):5–11

Huynh BC, Rovner A, Rich MW (2008) Identification of older patients with heart failure who may be candidates for hospice care: development of a simple four-item risk score. J Am Geri Soc 56:1111–1115

Johnson MJ (2007) Management of end stage cardiac failure. Postgra Med J 83:395–401

Levy WC, Mozaffarian D, Linker DT et al (2006) The Seattle heart failure model: prediction of survival in heart failure. Circulation 113:1424–1433

O'Conner CM, Abraham WT, Albert NM et al (2008) Predictors of mortality after discharge in patients hospitalized with heart failure: an analysis from the Organized Program to Initiate Lifesaving Treatment in Hospitalized Patients with Heart Failure (OPTIMIZE-HF). Am Heart J 156:662–673

Stuart B (2007) Palliative care and hospice in advanced heart failure. J Palliat Med 10:210–228

Wilkoff BL, Auricchio A, Brugada J et al (2008) HRS/EHRA expert consensus on the monitoring of cardiovascular implantable electronic devices (CIEDs): description of techniques, indications, personnel, frequency and ethical considerations. Europace 10:707–725

6 Pulmonary Palliative Care Issues

Karin B. Porter-Williamson

ABSTRACT

Determining patient-centered goals of care is important for facilitating a plan of care that makes sense to the patient, family, and health care providers. Serial therapeutic trials can be an important strategy in symptom management and, additionally, in determining reversibility of the patient's condition. An intervention can be considered palliative if it is capable of improving a symptom or quality of life and is fitting with the patient's goals. Dyspnea is an incapacitating symptom driven by many possible underlying factors and is associated with a high burden of suffering from associated depression, anxiety, and social isolation. Treatments for dyspnea are many, and include opioids, etiology-directed interventions which include breaking the dyspnea–anxiety–dyspnea cycle. An understanding of the pharmacokinetics of opioid medications is central to appropriate dosing and titration. Secretions at the end of life similarly require pharmacologic intervention.

Key Words: Dyspnea; Opioid medications; Anxiety; Depression; Pharmacokinetics; Symptom management; Palliative; Treatments

> *Mr. H is a 67-year-old male with advanced COPD and stage 4 non-small cell lung cancer which has progressed in spite of treatment with combination chemotherapy and radiation. He has been admitted to the hospital with rapidly worsening dyspnea and cough. On initial exam, the patient is breathing 33 times per minute, is using accessory muscles, can speak only short sentences, and appears panicked. Chest X-ray shows a right middle lobe infiltrate, compressive atelectasis, and a moderate size pleural effusion on the right side.*

From: *Current Clinical Oncology: Palliative Care: A Case-based Guide,*
Edited by: J.E. Loitman et al. DOI: 10.1007/978-1-60761-590-3_6,
© Springer Science+Business Media, LLC 2010

CONSIDER

1. The etiologic and pathophysiologic entities important in assessing pulmonary symptoms
2. The treatment modalities for the management of dyspnea
3. The primary teaching points for patients and families when starting opioid medications
4. The logic behind dosage and timing of opioid titration
5. Common techniques and medications to use for the management of secretions at end of life

KEY POINTS

- Determination of patient-centered goals of care is of primary importance for facilitating a plan of care which makes sense to the patient, family, and health care providers.
- Any intervention can be considered palliative if it is capable of improving a symptom or quality of life and is fitting with the patient's goals.
- Treatments for dyspnea are many and include opioids, etiology-directed interventions, as well as psychosocial support to help break the dyspnea–anxiety–dyspnea cycle.
- An understanding of the pharmacokinetics of opioid medications is central to appropriate dosing and titration.
- Dyspnea is an incapacitating symptom driven by many possible underlying factors and associated with a high burden of suffering from associated depression, anxiety, and social isolation.
- Serial therapeutic trials can be an important strategy in symptom management and, additionally, in determining reversibility of the patient's condition.

SCENARIO 1:
GOALS OF CARE DIRECT TREATMENT PLAN

> *Mr. H and his son are present for your initial evaluation, at which time it is necessary to make several important decisions about Mr. H's goals and expectations regarding his medical treatment. Mr. H appears to be at a fork in the road, his condition deteriorating rapidly into respiratory failure which may or may not be meaningfully reversible. You ask Mr. H what he understands of his illness and he replies that he knows the cancer cannot be cured; however, he is hoping that he will live to his 50th Anniversary, which is 3 years away. His son adds that Dad "has always been a fighter, so if there is anything that will help him live longer, he wants to try it, even if it means going on machines." You see the patient nodding in the background, gripping the rail on the bed as he breathes.*

Numerous conditions create the clinical picture of dyspnea and increased work of breathing: advanced lung cancer with potential compressive atelectasis from tumor, potential postobstructive pneumonia, an effusion which is either parapneumonic or malignant and contributing symptomatology from advanced COPD. Some of these contributors are irreversible, and some may potentially be altered with intervention. Mr. H's treatment goals include an aggressive trial of intervention for the reversible conditions, including intubation if necessary, but his expectations regarding the outcome of such treatment and his condition are not realistic. Fear or anxiety regarding dyspnea or death can drive both the decision-making and the dyspnea. Nonetheless, immediate global treatment considerations must be addressed, such as the need for artificial life support, either in the form of Bi-PAP or intubation and mechanical ventilation, and immediate institution of symptom management strategies to decrease the distress of the dyspnea.

Disease-directed interventions

Contributors to dyspnea and cough in our patient	Treatment options
Mechanical airway compression	Endoscopic stent placement
Pneumonia	Antibiotics
Malignant effusion	Thoracentesis, talc pleurodesis, placement of pleurovac drain
COPD/airway reactivity	O2, steroids, bronchodilators
Other contributors to consider	
Pulmonary embolism	Anticoagulation
Congestive heart failure	Diuretics, ace-inhibitors, beta blockers
Anemia	Transfusion, erythropoetin
Carcinomatous lymphangitis	Corticosteroids, chemotherapy
Pericardial effusion	Pericardiocentesis, pericardial window
Radiation pneumonitis	Corticosteroids
Pneumothorax	Chest tube

In helping patients and families weigh their options, it is important to clearly outline the treatment options, with their potential benefits and burdens. These benefits and burdens need to be considered in light of the overall goal of care. Treatment directed at the underlying etiology will provide added meaningful benefit for the patient, if that treatment fits with the patient's goal of care and overall condition *(1)*. Disease modifying therapies may not be possible or the burden may not fit the patient's goal of care. Interventions should be determined based on the goal of care, feasibility, and indication. Symptoms should be modified regardless of the goal of care. (For more on Goals of Care, see Chap. 1.)

SCENARIO 2:
OPIOIDS FOR DYSPNEA

Mr. H and his son feel strongly that a trial of Bi-PAP be instituted. Antibiotics, nebulizers, steroids, and prn morphine are implemented. A thoracentesis is performed to help reduce the work of breathing. Over the next few days the patient feels better and is able to take breaks from the Bi-PAP for several hours at a time. A bronchoscopy reveals an endobronchial lesion which is stented. The pleural fluid cytology comes back positive for poorly differentiated adenocarcinoma, and the patient's oncologist tells the patient and his wife that no more chemotherapy can be offered. The patient continues to have a chronic baseline dyspnea with bouts of worsening dyspnea, cough, and anxiety, especially if he exerts himself at all or is off of the Bi-PAP for too long. Your review of the patient's medications reveals that he has not been using the prn morphine. On questioning, the patient states that it is because he has heard that morphine is what they use "to put you out in the end."

Studies show that when opioids are dosed logically and titration monitored carefully, the risks of respiratory depression are largely mitigated. In a study of 31 patients with advanced cancer and lung disease receiving doses of morphine as high as 90 mg/day, no significant differences were seen in respiratory rate, ABG values, or peak flow rates. The authors concluded that systemic oral morphine is safe and efficacious in the majority of those with advanced cancer with concomitant respiratory disease (2). Care should be taken in the opioid naïve patient to "start low and go slow"; however, the concern for respiratory depression should not preclude administration of these medications for symptom relief. Other common side effects of opioids including drowsiness and nausea will attenuate after a few days of medication administration. It can be helpful to explain to patients and families when starting an opioid for pain or dyspnea management that it would be normal for the patient to be sleepier, not only as a side effect of the medication but also because the patient may finally be able to rest once comfortable enough for restorative sleep.

In treating dyspnea, opioids work at both the peripheral and central nervous system levels, via suppression of opioid receptors located in the lung parenchyma (juxtapulmonary receptors in the alveoli), stretch and chemical irritant receptors in the airway, and central receptors in the spinal cord and respiratory centers. While morphine is the drug most commonly suggested, any Mu receptor agonist should be effective in treating the symptom. In general, lower doses of medication may be needed to provide relief from dyspnea when compared with doses needed to manage pain and is certainly a patient-specific determination. The right dose of medication for the patient is that which controls the symptom with an acceptable side-effect profile. No more, no less. There is no ceiling on the amount of medication that can be given. Telling patients and families about these "opioid pearls" can help to alleviate fears of being "put out" as well as fears that they must use their medications sparingly so that they will not reach "the limit" and be told they can have no more.

When a patient is experiencing a continuous symptom, initiate a scheduled ongoing medication to address the symptom. The dosing schedule should be based at the half-life of the drug, and the as-needed (prn) doses should be based on the Tmax of the drug, which is the time that it takes the medication to reach its maximal concentration in the blood after the dose is given. For oral morphine, oxycodone, and hydromorphone, the half-life is 4 h and the Tmax is 60–90 min whereas the Tmax for an intravenous dose is 10–15 min. One can consider a longer interval for the prn dose for the elderly patient or those with liver/kidney dysfunction. The appropriate amount of opioid for the prn dose should be 5–15% of the patient's 24-h opioid dose. For our opioid naïve patient, one should consider starting a low dose, immediate release opioid around the clock, with breakthrough medication provided every 60–90 min as needed. Once the patient has symptom relief on a stable 24-h dose of medication, the patient can be transitioned to an equivalent dose of long-acting preparation, again with breakthrough medication provided at the Tmax of the drug. The following table outlines dosing strategies for two different patients with dyspnea, one who is opioid naïve and one who is not.

Patient type	Starting scheduled dose	Starting PRN dose	Day 3 evaluation – stable 24-h opioid use with relief	Next medication recommendation
Opioid naïve	MS-IR 2.5–5 mg q 4 h scheduled	MS-IR 2.5–5 mg q 1 h PRN	65 mg PO morphinetotal	MS-ER 30 mg; MS-IR 5–10 mg q1 h PRN dyspnea
Opioid Tolerant (60 mg/day MS-IR)	MS-ER 30 mg bid	MS-IR 5–10 mg q 1 h PRN	100 mg po morphinetotal	MS-ER 45 mg bid; MS-IR 5–15 mg PRN q1 h prn dyspnea

MS-IR = immediate release morphine sulfate
MS-ER = extended release morphine sulfate

SCENARIO 3:
MOOD AND DYSPNEA

A few more days have passed and the patient has recognized that "everything" is being done for him that may possibly be helpful and has decided that if he should deteriorate in spite of these treatments he no longer wishes to go onto the ventilator but would rather shift to a purely comfort-directed approach. His physical symptoms are better controlled and now his main anxiety revolves around his wife's difficulty handling his illness and impending death, as well as his own feelings of sadness and regret, feeling that he is letting them down. When he even thinks of his family he starts to have more difficulty breathing. He asks what you can do to help.

There is a strong association of depression and dyspnea, with both symptoms affecting up to 50% of patients with advanced COPD. Treating depression may actually be more beneficial in reducing anxiety than the use of benzodiazepines. Newer antidepressant agents that work through a combination of norepinephrine and serotonin reuptake inhibition have properties that may effectively address both depression and anxiety, making them an appropriate choice for our patient. One must bear in mind that antidepressant medications can take weeks to begin to work. Because the prevalence of clinically significant depression is reported as high as 75% in patients with advanced and life-threatening conditions, early and repeated assessment for depression is important for timely initiation of treatment *(3)*. If a prognosis of days to a few weeks does not afford the time for titration of a traditional antidepressant, one can consider the use of a stimulant agent such as methylphenidate or modafinil instead, as these agents begin to work in a much shorter period of time. Side effects that should be considered with these medications include anxiety, agitation, and delirium, and so may not be the best choice for a patient already dealing with anxiety. (For more on Psychiatric Issues, see Chap. 4.)

Anxiolytics have not been proven efficacious in the treatment of dyspnea. They may be considered if the patient has acute situational anxiety. A common, vicious cycle of anxiety and dyspnea has been recognized by qualitative studies of patients dealing with advanced lung disease. Patients become anxious for any number of reasons, followed by changes in their breathing patterns which in turn affect the mechanics of ventilation. If not disrupted, this cycle can become debilitating and can generate more dyspnea, and consequently more anxiety. Interventions which can help to break this cycle include providing a medical contact for the patient at home to provide reassurance, take vital signs or provide O2 and nebulizer treatments or walk the patient through an "exacerbation action plan." In addition, if consistent with the goals of care and the patients' prognosis, pulmonary rehabilitation programs which include patient self management education help patients develop self management skills that can be used in the face of mounting anxiety and dyspnea *(4)*.

One should also consider that the patient's anxiety may be related to unresolved family issues or a need for open communication amongst family about condition, prognosis, planning for the future, legacy building, completion of tasks to assure security for the family after his death, etc. Counseling for the patient and family plays a critical role in relieving symptoms in addition to pharmacologic intervention. (For more on Communication, see Chap. 2.)

SCENARIO 4:
SECRETIONS AT THE END OF LIFE

Mr. H continues to make slow improvements in his respiratory function over the next few days and starts to talk about wanting to be at home. He is now free from the Bi-PAP, though he continues to need several liters of oxygen. He is discharged home with hospice care to achieve symptom relief as the primary goal of care. Two weeks after he gets home, you do a follow-up home visit. The patient has become much more lethargic over the last 2 days and has developed "a rattle." The family wants to suction the patient because they are afraid he "is drowning." Your examination of his chest reveals recurrent dullness on the right side to percussion. Overall, the patient appears to be comfortable though he appears to be in the active dying process. The family is anxious to know what they should be doing to make him more comfortable and would like to increase his scheduled concentrated oral morphine, though he has needed only a few prn doses each day.

The patient's condition and the goals of care have evolved over time. While it is likely that the malignant effusion has recurred, his goal of care is comfort and to remain at home so a thoracentesis would not be indicated. Given that the patient is comfortable in appearance on the current medication regimen, family support and education is indicated. In an attempt to minimize fluids in the oral cavity that could potentially contribute to the secretions, one could consider, converting the oral morphine to either suppository form or to a transdermal fentanyl preparation. Typically, patients in this state are mouth breathing, so, regular oral care or a trial of intermittent postural drainage to physically move the secretions may reduce the patient's rattle. Anticholinergic agents prevent secretion production and help the noise and family suffering from hearing the rattle. Scopolamine patches are easy though they take approximately 24 h to have an effect. Atropine eye drops administered sublingually have a more rapid onset of action and are easy to administer. Oral medications such as glycopyrrolate and hyoscyamine are also efficacious. Suctioning the patient will likely cause the patient more discomfort, will likely cause the patient's airway to generate even more secretions, and will likely not be effective, as most of the secretions are lower in the airway than a suction catheter can reach. (For more on last hours, see Chap. 10.)

REFERENCES

1. Del Fabbro E, Dalal S, Bruera E (2006) Symptom control in palliative care – Part III: dyspnea and delirium. J Palliat Med 9(2):422–436
2. Walsh TD, Rivera NI, Kaiko R (2003) Oral morphine and respiratory function amongst hospice inpatients with advanced cancer. Support Care Cancer 11(12):780–784
3. Noorani NH, Montagnini M (2007) Recognizing depression in palliative care patients. J Palliat Med 10(2):458–464
4. Rocker GM, Sinuff T, Horton R, Hernandez P (2007) Advanced chronic obstructive pulmonary disease: innovative approaches to palliation. J Palliat Med 10(3):783–797

7

GI Palliative Care Issues

Eric Roeland and Gary Buckholz

ABSTRACT

The physician should always consider the etiology and pathophysiology of constipation, nausea, and vomiting before starting treatment. The work up and treatment for the symptom of abdominal pain includes a digital rectal exam for complete assessment of constipation and diarrhea. A plain abdominal radiograph is an inexpensive and useful tool for this type of evaluation. Stimulant laxatives are the treatment of choice for opioid-induced constipation. Pain at the end of life is often treated with opioid analgesics which are consequently associated with GI issues. Opioids cause constipation for which tolerance does not occur and requires prophylaxis. Fiber or other bulk forming laxatives can worsen opioid-induced constipation. Additional symptoms or problems that might develop related to abdominal pain include pseudodiarrhea.

Key Words: Constipation; Bowel obstruction; Nausea; Nasogastric tube; Bowel; Abdominal pain; Opioids; Laxatives; Diarrhea; Prophylaxis; Abdominal radiograph

> *Mrs. C is a 43-year-old woman diagnosed with ovarian cancer 1 year ago. She underwent a tumor debulking procedure and adjuvant chemotherapy and had a few months without events. For several weeks, she has been experiencing diffuse lower abdominal pain which she describes as a 5/10, constant, crampy, dull ache. She is presumed to have adhesions from surgery so her primary physician starts her on an oral opioid regimen for pain.*

CONSIDER

1. The GI issues associated with starting patients on opioids for pain
2. The work up and treatment for the symptom of abdominal pain
3. Additional symptoms or problems that might develop related to abdominal pain

From: *Current Clinical Oncology: Palliative Care: A Case-based Guide,*
Edited by: J.E. Loitman et al. DOI: 10.1007/978-1-60761-590-3_7,
© Springer Science + Business Media, LLC 2010

KEY POINTS

- Individual variation is an essential component in the evaluation of constipation.
- A complete assessment of constipation and diarrhea requires a digital rectal exam.
- A plain abdominal radiograph is an inexpensive and useful tool for the evaluation of constipation and diarrhea.
- Opioids cause constipation for which tolerance does not occur and requires prophylaxis.
- Stimulant laxatives are the treatment of choice for opioid-induced constipation.
- Fiber or other bulk forming laxatives can worsen opioid-induced constipation.
- Pseudodiarrhea can occur in the setting of constipation.
- Always consider the etiology and pathophysiology of nausea and vomiting before starting treatment.
- Anticipatory nausea is the feeling of nausea associated with the thought of past nausea provoking experiences.
- In the setting of malignant bowel obstruction, the use of octreotide may avert the need for nasogastric tube placement to decompress the bowel.

SCENARIO 1:
OPIOID-INDUCED CONSTIPATION

> *Mrs. C reports opioids previously worked well. She is concerned about the lack of effect on her abdominal pain now. In the last week, her pain has increased to 10/10 while walking or trying to move her bowels. Upon further questioning, she reports that she has not "had a good bowel movement in one week."*

Constipation is defined as difficult defecation with reduced number of bowel movements experienced outside the normal elimination patterns of an individual. Constipation causes considerable discomfort and suffering for patients. A proper constipation history includes more than simply asking when a patient's last bowel movement occurred. Clinicians must inquire regarding changes from the patient's normal stool pattern and characteristics of the stool over time. Although opioids are a very common cause of constipation, a thorough history should include information regarding other potential causes of constipation including: altered diet (dehydration, decreased oral intake), decreased physical activity, medications (5-HT3 receptor antagonists, calcium or aluminum-containing antacids, calcium channel blockers, anticholinergics, iron, and chemotherapeutic agents), mechanical obstruction (intrinsic or extrinsic compression by masses or adhesions), motility/neurologic disorders (autonomic failure, spinal cord lesions, tumor invasion of nerves), and endocrine/metabolic disorders (hypercalcemia, hypokalemia, diabetes, hypothyroidism). While several etiologies may apply to Mrs. C's constipation, this section will focus on opioid-induced constipation. Opioids primarily cause constipation by binding to mu-opioid receptors present on enteric neurons disrupting neural coordination necessary for peristalsis, which slows down bowel motility.

The physical exam for a patient with constipation should focus on the basics of the abdominal exam including: observation, auscultation, palpation, and percussion. Observe any visible masses, abdominal distension, or scars. Absence of or decreased bowel sounds is associated with ileus; high-pitched or hyperactive bowel sounds are present with obstruction. A complete physical exam includes a digital rectal exam noting rectal tone, hemorrhoids, fissures, scaring, tumor, rectal prolapse, and the presence/characteristics of stool in the rectal vault.

Table 1
Opioid-induced constipation prophylaxis

Prophylactic interventions	Examples
1. Stimulant laxatives	Senna/bisacodyl
	(Senna is available in a formulation with docusate 100 mg)
2. Osmotic laxatives	Polyethylene glycol, lactulose, sorbitol, magnesium hydroxide
3. Prokinetic agents	Metoclopramide, erythromycin

Table 2
Therapeutic constipation interventions

Therapeutic interventions	Examples
Stimulant suppository	Biscacodyl
Enema	Water, fleets phosphosoda, mineral oil
Oral osmotic agents	Polyethylene glycol, lactulose, sorbitol, magnesium hydroxide
Peripheral acting mu-receptor antagonists	Methylnaltrexone (SQ/IV only) Alvimopan (PO only)

The workup of constipation may include a plain abdominal radiograph or laboratory tests if the goals of care or potential interventions warrant such. Noting stool and gas pattern, presence of air-fluid levels, and dilated loops of bowel help determine the cause of constipation. Altered potassium, calcium, and thyroid-stimulating hormone levels may contribute to constipation and if suspected, appropriate labs should be drawn.

Treatment of opioid-induced constipation includes both prophylaxis and therapeutic treatment of acute constipation. Since opioids have the unintended consequence of slowing bowel motility and drying stool, prophylaxis should begin at the initiation of an opioid regimen. Stool softeners such as docusate are frequently implemented in conjunction with a laxative. Laxative prophylaxis (Table 1) can be approached in a stepwise additive fashion (1 then 1 + 2, then 1 + 2 + 3). Fiber or other bulk forming laxatives can worsen opioid-induced constipation.

The treatment choice for acute constipation depends on the history and physical exam findings. For example, if the patient has either soft stool or the absence of stool in the rectal vault, a stimulant suppository is recommended. If the physical exam reveals hard stool in the rectal vault, an enema would be the intervention of choice. In some cases, manual disimpaction may be necessary. If there is no stool in the rectal vault, but the abdominal plain film reveals high impaction, then a tap water enema may alleviate symptoms. Table 2 lists therapeutic constipation interventions.

SCENARIO 2:
DIARRHEA IN THE SETTING OF CONSTIPATION

Mrs. C has continued her opioid regimen for abdominal pain and has been diligent about taking her prescribed laxatives. However, over the last 2 days she started having uncontrolled diarrhea and increased abdominal discomfort. She took one dose of loperamide and wonders if she should cut back on her laxatives.

Diarrhea is generally defined as frequent loose or liquid bowel movements. A careful history and physical exam is necessary to determine the likely etiology. The history should include onset, frequency, approximate volume, presence or absence of blood, and other characteristics of the stool. It is important to classify diarrhea as acute (<2 weeks), persistent (2–4 weeks), or chronic (>4 weeks). Complete abdominal exam, digital rectal exam, temperature, and assessment of hydration status are helpful. History and exam will guide potential diagnostic evaluations, which might include stool studies for chemical and microbiological analysis as well as occult blood testing. Bloodwork may help evaluate hydration status and evidence of leukocytosis may suggest an infectious etiology. Therapies for treating diarrhea should target the underlying cause. Since death from diarrhea is often secondary to dehydration, appropriate rehydration and replacement of lost electrolytes is important and will help patients feel better. Antidiarrheal agents such as loperamide can help decrease stool frequency, but may prolong some infectious etiologies.

In otherwise healthy individuals, acute diarrhea is often infectious (viral, bacteria, or parasitic). For patients with advanced chronic illness, *Clostridium difficile* should be considered especially after a recent hospitalization and/or antibiotic use. For patients on opioids, diarrhea associated with laxative use and pseudodiarrhea, the passage of loose stool around a fecal impaction, is common and should be considered. Impaction in the face of persistent loose stools is evaluated with a digital rectal exam. A plain radiograph of the abdomen showing stool pattern with evidence of inspisated stool in the colon or rectal vault can help to diagnose pseudodiarrhea. Clinicians should generally refrain from prescribing antidiarrheal agents to patients on opioids and laxatives. Many are available over-the-counter and may worsen diarrhea associated with fecal impaction. Counsel patients who are taking opioids and laxatives to call prior to purchasing over-the-counter antidiarrheal medications.

SCENARIO 3:
DEVELOPMENT OF NAUSEA AND EMESIS

> *Mrs. C calls you reporting that her pain and diarrhea are well controlled, but she has worsening nausea and vomiting. She feels nauseous even "at the site of her favorite food" and vomits roughly four times a week. She still has flatus and her last bowel movement was yesterday. She asks if there is anything you can do to help her control her nausea.*

Nausea is the unpleasant sensation for the need to vomit associated with autonomic symptoms, including cold sweats, tachycardia, diarrhea, and pallor. Nausea and vomiting reduce patients' quality of life and affect their compliance to therapy. The cause of each patient's symptoms may differ and an accurate evaluation is crucial for the treatment of the symptom. One helpful way to consider the differential diagnosis of nausea is the 12 Ms (Table 3).

In addition to a careful history, examination, and review of medications, treating nausea requires an understanding of the pathophysiology. Treating the cause of nausea allows you to customize treatment to meet each patient's needs. To simplify our approach, it is easiest to breakdown nausea into two anatomical locations: the brain and the gastrointestinal (GI) tract. The brain has roughly five areas that modulate the perception of nausea including: the

Table 3
12 Ms of emesis

12 "Ms" of emesis	
Metastases	Mechanical obstruction
Meningeal irritation	Motility
Movement	Metabolic
Mentation (e.g., anxiety)	Microbes (infection)
Medications	Myocardial
Mucosal irritation	Maternity

Table 4
Choosing appropriate antiemetics based on responsible neurotransmitters

Anatomical location	Neurotransmitter	Example drugs
Cortex	Unclear	Dexamethasone, lorazepam, THC
Chemoreceptor	Dopamine	Haloperidol, metoclopramide, prochlorperazine
trigger zone	Serotonin	Ondansetron, granisetron
Vomiting center	Histamine	Diphenhydramine, meclizine, hydroxyzine
	Acetylcholine	Scopolamine
Vestibular apparatus	Histamine	Diphenhydramine, meclizine, hydroxyzine
	Acetylcholine	Scopolamine

cortex, fourth ventricle (chemoreceptor trigger zone), brainstem, medulla (vomiting center), and vestibular apparatus. Increased intracranial pressure in the cortex or the medulla secondary to vascular lesions, neoplasm, and/or inflammation induces nausea; medications, toxins, and electrolyte disturbances stimulate the chemoreceptor trigger zone; infection, motion, or benign positional vertigo may stimulate the vestibular apparatus.

In the GI tract, obstruction, motility disorders, gastric atony, infection, and even constipation may be the cause of nausea. When constipation is the etiology, aggressive use of laxatives are indicated to relieve both symptoms of nausea and constipation. In the setting of bowel distension, chemotherapy, or radiation therapy, the enterochromaffin cells of the GI tract stimulate emesis via the release of serotonin and stimulation of the vagus nerve. There is good evidence to support using 5HT-3 antagonists such as ondansetron for prophylaxis of radiation or chemotherapy-induced nausea.

When a patient experiences chronic and/or intense nausea/vomiting, they may develop anticipatory nausea, which is the phenomenon of feeling nauseous at the thought of or in association with previously experienced nausea. Nonpharmacologic measures and benzodiazepines are used to treat the subsequent anxiety and can decrease the feeling of nausea (Table 4).

When treating nausea, symptomatically, conceptualize the likely underlying pathology and neurotransmitters involved. Choose an agent from one drug class and titrate to effect or side effect. Add and titrate additional agents with different mechanisms of action if needed.

For severe nausea, consider starting multiple agents associated with different mechanisms of action at the same time again guided by the likely differential and pathophysiology. Once the symptom is controlled, decrease doses of medication to the lowest effective dose and discontinue medications when possible. These strategies allow for quick symptom control and avoidance of polypharmacy and associated adverse effects.

SCENARIO 4:
PALLIATION OF INOPERABLE BOWEL OBSTRUCTION

Mrs. C's opioid-induced constipation improves on her new bowel regimen. She does very well until 1 year later when she presents with bloating, nausea, vomiting, and intense, 8/10 crampy abdominal pain. She is unable to take her oral medications. She is diagnosed with a malignant bowel obstruction and recurrent disease. She is neither a candidate for surgery nor stent placement. Medical management of her symptoms is essential for quality of life.

In general, malignant bowel obstruction (MBO) results from three mechanisms including: extrinsic compression from tumor masses or adhesions, intraluminal compression from a growing tumor, or intramural tumor growth causing disruption of normal bowel peristalsis. Other factors also contribute to the formation of MBO including constipating drugs (as discussed above), fecal impaction, and inflammation.

MBO is a frequent cancer complication seen in ovarian and colon cancer. Treatment options begin with nasograstric tubes, intravenous fluids, and assessment for surgical debulking or palliation with a venting gastrostomy tube or a metallic stent across the obstructed site(s). Many patients like Mrs. C are not eligible for surgical options given the surgical risks, poor performance status, multiple obstruction sites, and limited prognosis. In such circumstances, hospice should be considered if not already instituted. Regardless, medical management consists of a combination of parenteral opioids, antispasmodics, antiemetics, corticosteroids, anticholineric agents, antisecretory hormones, and intravenous fluids. Venting gastrostomies are frequently utilized in conjunction with medical management to decompress gas and fluid build-up of the intestines.

Octreotide can be utilized to decrease intestinal fluid volume and decrease colicky pain. Octreotide mimics the effect of somatostatin and functions as a neurohormone inhibiting the glandular secretions of growth hormone, thyroid-stimulating hormone, adrenocortitropin hormone, and prolactin; it also decreases the release of gastrin, insulin, glucagon, gastric acid, pancreatic enzymes, and cholecystokinin. Octreotide reduces neurotransmission in the peripheral nerves of the GI tract causing decreased peristalsis and splanchnic blood flow. This may produce a medical "decompression" of the bowel and allow discontinuation or avoidance of a nasogastric tube which is uncomfortable (Table 5).

Table 5
Commonly used medications

Medication	Indication	Initial dose	Common maximum adult dosing
Stool softener			
Docusate sodium	Constipation	100 mg	500 mg BID [a]
Stimulant laxative			
Senna	Constipation	8.6 mg (1 tablet)	34.4 mg (4 tablets) BID
Bisacodyl	Constipation	10 mg	15 mg/dose PO or 10 mg/dose PR
Osmotic laxative			
Polyethylene glycol	Constipation	17 g	34 g/day
Lactulose	Constipation	30 ml	45 ml TID-QID
Sorbitol	Constipation	30 ml	30 ml Q6 h [a]
Magnesium hydroxide	Constipation	20 ml	80 ml daily
Prokinetic agent & antiemetic			
Metoclopramide	Constipation, nausea	10 mg	45 mg/day or 15 mg per single dose
Erythromycin	Constipation, nausea	150 mg	250 mg QID
Enema			
Fleet Phosphosoda Enema	Constipation	1 bottle (118 ml)	1 bottle (118 ml) daily
Benzodiazepine			
Lorazepam	Nausea/emesis	0.5 mg	2 mg Q4 h as needed [a]
Dopamine antagonist			
Haloperidol	Nausea/emesis	0.5 mg	8 mg total daily [a]
Prochlorperazine maleate	Nausea/emesis	5 mg	10 mg QID
5-HT3 receptor antagonist			
Ondansetron	Nausea/emesis	4 mg	24 mg total daily
Antihistamine			
Diphenhydramine	Nausea/emesis	25 mg	300 mg total daily
Meclizine	Nausea/emesis	25 mg	50 mg total daily
Hydroxyzine	Nausea/emesis	25 mg	400 mg total daily

[a]Based on expert opinion

FURTHER READING

Bruera E, Fadul N (2006) Constipation and diarrhea. In: Bruera E, Higginson IJ, Ripamonti C, von Gunten CF (eds) Textbook of palliative medicine, 1st edn. Oxford University Press, New York, NY, pp 554–570

Jatoi A, Podratz KC, Gill P et al (2004) Pathophysiology and palliation of inoperable bowel obstruction in patients with ovarian cancer. J Support Oncol 2(4): 323–334; discussion 334

Muir JC, von Gunten CF (2000) Antisecretory agents in gastrointestinal obstruction. Clin Geriatr Med 16(2):327–334

Thomas J (2007) Cancer-related constipation. Curr Oncol Rep 9(4):278–284

8 Palliative Pain Issues

Miles J. Belgrade

ABSTRACT

Pain often presents with a very complex mixture of medical, psychological, and social factors. Physicians frequently approach persistent pain with apprehension and biases. Patients and families often believe pain can be cured, while clinical medicine is still far from cure or even consistent success. This chapter outlines an approach that allows physicians to be dispassionate about the process of pain management, yet compassionate for their patients in pain. It presents a strategy and framework for understanding and approaching patients with advanced medical illness who have complex pain issues. Through a discussion of the overall goals of therapy relative to pain relief goals, this approach helps physicians and their patients determine the actual or inferred pathophysiology of pain, the contributing factors that impact the pain experience, and the numerous barriers that complicate pain assessments and treatment. Utilization of opioid analgesics, adjuvants, and nonpharmacologic are also incorporated into this model.

Key Words: Opioid analgesics; Pain assessment; Pain treatment; Pathophysiology of pain; Pain management

Ms. N is a 27-year-old female with systemic lupus erythematosis and renal osteodystrophy with a history of multiple fractures and mechanical abnormalities contributing to multiregional joint, bone, and muscular pain. She is on chronic hemodialysis for end-stage renal disease. She has chronic pain in her shoulders, back, hips, and both legs in addition to daily headaches. She has severe hearing impairment and is blind in one eye from infection.

She lives with her mother, sister, and niece and spends most of her time at home watching television. She receives social security disability income. Communication is also difficult because she is hostile toward the clinicians. She has been unreliable with adhering to physician recommendations in the past.

From: *Current Clinical Oncology: Palliative Care: A Case-based Guide,*
Edited by: J.E. Loitman et al. DOI: 10.1007/978-1-60761-590-3_8,
© Springer Science+Business Media, LLC 2010

CONSIDER

1. A strategy and framework for understanding and approaching patients with advanced medical illness who have complex pain issues
2. An approach allowing physicians to be *dispassionate* about the process of pain management, yet *compassionate* for their patients in pain
3. A discussion related to overall goals of therapy relative to pain relief goals

KEY POINTS

- Pain often presents with a very complex mixture of medical, psychological, and social factors. Physicians frequently approach persistent pain with apprehension and biases. Our training leaves us ill-prepared to deal with it.
- Patients and families often believe pain can be cured, while medical science is still far from cure or even consistent success.
- Pain issues are similar regardless of the proximity to the end of life.
- Determining the actual or inferred pathophysiology of pain directs treatment options.
- Contributing factors impact the pain experience.
- Numerous barriers complicate pain assessments and treatment.

SCENARIO 1:
GOALS OF THERAPY

Ms. N's primary physician prescribes hydrocodone/acetaminophen 5 mg/500 mg every 4 h as needed. She says she takes about six to eight tablets per day but it is not controlling the pain. The physician suspects she is abusing opioids because of lost prescriptions and requests for early prescriptions and for "something stronger." She uses doses of hydroxyzine for uncontrolled itching regularly. She had previously tried nonsteroidal antiinflammatory drugs (NSAIDs), antidepressants, and diazepam without relief. She tried biofeedback, chiropractic care, and counseling, but she is currently only utilizing medications. She has moderate lip reading ability and limited hearing. Her mother is present and appears to be an exhausted caregiver and advocate.

Many elements above make managing her pain challenging. Frustration occurs when pain is widespread or communication is made difficult due to hearing loss and personality. Efforts to provide stable analgesia may be sabotaged by a loss of control over the prescription process or by a condition that may be progressive with an unpredictable, ill-defined timeline.

Developing a pain management strategy begins with determining the goals of care regarding pain. The physician collaborates with the patient on the goals of care and the treatment strategy. The healthcare provider must provide an estimated prognosis to patients such that goals are concordant with planned therapies (Fig. 1). The choice of palliative vs. restorative treatment goals for persistent pain is influenced by disease burden, the level of responsibility a patient accepts, and what level of treatment-related risk is appropriate. The goals and treatments are different for a healthy patient with an ankle sprain than for a patient with uncontrolled ankle pain due to Charcot joint with recurrent infection, underlying diabetes, and renal failure. Where does Ms. N fit on the chart in Fig. 1 below?

Goals of Pain Management in Palliative Care vs. Chronic Pain

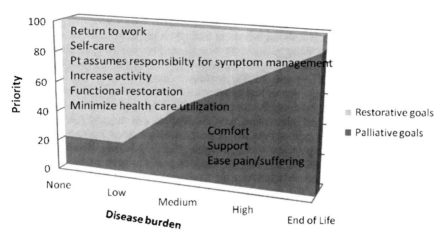

Fig. 1. Priority for pain management goals depends on the degree of disease burden.

SCENARIO 2:
THE PATHOPHYSIOLOGIC TYPES OF PAIN

> *On physical examination, Ms. N presents as a young woman of short stature, her physician has to repeat things over and over before she understands. She is completely blind in the right eye. Her skin is excoriated in places where she scratches. There are deformities of the long bones at sites of healed old fractures. She has multiple tender points on the neck, back, and limbs. She can walk independently. She has peripheral neuropathy with a stocking distribution loss of pinprick and vibratory senses and absent deep tendon reflexes.*

Ms. N is not near the end of life, but her disease is disabling and life-limiting. Providing aggressive pain management, including opioid analgesics, should be balanced with structuring the treatment so that the prescribing process is more successful and less prone to failure. Her disease burden is high, dictating a treatment approach that is more palliative. Incorporating aggressive rehabilitation or physical reconditioning is more appropriate for patients with low disease burden. Establishing the level of disease burden helps guide the clinical approach.

Pain science has advanced in the last two decades allowing identification of different pathophysiologic mechanisms for discrete types of pain. *Nociceptive pain* is due to activation of nociceptors either through mechanical compression or by inflammation. *Neuropathic pain* occurs with damage or dysfunction to the peripheral or central nervous system. *Bone pain* can be caused by osteoclast activity as in bone metastases; pain is maintained by activated glial cells in the spinal cord. *Muscular pain* has its own mechanisms that are distinct from the others. These four pain types respond to different therapeutic interventions by virtue of their distinct mechanisms. NSAIDs are used for inflammatory pain, whereas mechanical pain is generally treated with specific measures to decompress or stabilize involved structures.

Examples include vertebroplasty in spinal compression fracture, bracing, debulking a mass, and draining an effusion. For neuropathic pain, hyperexcitable and sensitized neurons are targeted for pain therapies. Gabapentin, an anticonvulsant, regulates neuronal hyperactivity by modulating the voltage-gated calcium channels located on the nerves. Tricyclic antidepressants affect the descending modulation of pain through serotonin and norepinephrine reuptake inhibition in the brainstem. Muscular pain typically requires physical therapeutic approaches like stretching, range of motion, TENS, massage, aquatic therapy, and mobilization. Sometimes trigger point injection or botulinum toxin injections are used to break a cycle of muscle dysfunction. Bone pain responds to prostaglandin inhibitors or corticosteroids.

On the basis of historical information, pain distribution, and physical findings, one can infer the pathophysiologic type of pain. Ms. N presents with three of the four cardinal pain types: bone pain, muscular pain, and nociceptive pain (Fig. 2). A history of multiple fractures underlying renal osteodystrophy and bone deformities points to bone pain as an important mechanism. Muscular pain is inferred from the tenderness on exam. Lupus predisposes her to inflammatory joint pain. The presence of neuropathy suggests neuropathic pain, but her symptoms do not correlate anatomically (e.g., no burning pain in a stocking distribution).

With three inferred pain types, the next step in a pain management strategy is selecting medications and other treatments. An antiinflammatory drug would reduce nociceptive pain from lupus arthritis. NSAIDs would also help manage bone pain due to fracture and microfractures which may continue to occur. Muscle pain is generally managed with physical modalities that could include stretching, posture correction, exercise, local modalities like ultrasound, passive range of motion, trigger point injection, and muscle relaxants. Table 1 summarizes the pain types and some of the specific treatment strategies for those pain types.

| Nociceptive | Muscle |
★	★
Neuropathic	Bone
	★

Fig. 2. Check off grid for noting physiologic types of pain.

Table 1
Physiological types of pain and their associated treatment strategies

Type of pain	Treatment strategies
Nociceptive	NSAID, corticosteroid, mechanical decompression/stabilization
Neuropathic	Anticonvulsants (gabapentin, pregabalin) antidepressants (Tricyclic, SNRIs)
Muscle	Physical therapies, muscle relaxants, trigger point injections
Bone	NSAID, corticosteroid, calcitonin, bisphosphonates

SCENARIO 3:
CONTRIBUTING FACTORS AND BARRIERS

Ms. N's fragile bone status is an important primary cause of her pain. Ms. N may be avoiding activities that take her out of the house because pain is worse with standing or walking. Hearing and visual impairment are hampering communication with Ms. N. Her anger and lack of trust interferes with her receptivity toward recommended treatments and engenders a hands-off approach by many clinicians.

Contributing factors amplify pain or perpetuate it but are not the original cause of pain. For example, pain from a simple rib fracture is amplified with coughing from bronchitis. Managing contributing factors will lessen pain. Treating the cough will reduce the amplified pain from a rib fracture. Other contributing factors include anxiety, depression, fever, poor positioning, weight-bearing on an unstable joint, edema in a painful limb, and vomiting in a patient with back or abdominal pain. Often, an improvement in pain control is achieved when contributing factors are modified, even when the underlying pain is intractable. Treatment of osteodystrophy and functional activities like walking and climbing stairs limit fracture risk and reduce pain exacerbation. Physical or occupational therapy evaluation can ameliorate pain in the hips and lower limbs by reducing weight-bearing forces with assistive devices like a cane or walker.

Barriers neither cause nor amplify the pain, but do make assessment or management more difficult. Insurance noncoverage for effective pain treatments has become an increasingly important hinderance to pain control. Language, cultural, and other communication barriers limit the ability to fully assess pain. Patient-centered factors such as low motivation, poor compliance, and chemical dependency may also impede ideal pain management. Such barriers are important to identify to better understand successes and failures of pain management strategies. Recognizing barriers may prevent continued escalation of ineffective therapies in a futile attempt to obtain relief and putting the patient at greater risk. Some barriers, once identified, can be effectively managed, thereby allowing pain management to take place with greater success.

Nonadherence with medication is an important barrier to providing aggressive pharmacological treatment for pain. Recognizing this, as a barrier, improves clinical management. One strategy includes frequent visits every 1 or 2 weeks. This provides a structure for the scheduled medications, which reduces the risk of misuse. Additionally, patients may feel more comfortable that the clinician is providing a more aggressive pain medicine approach.

SCENARIO 4:
MANAGING OPIOIDS

Because of Ms. N's compelling burden of disease, her physician decides to utilize opioid analgesics. The concerns about which opioid to choose and in what formulation are considered.

Table 2
Commonly used opioids with prolonged effects

Opioid	Dosages available	Dosing interval (default underlined)	Comments
Morphine	15, 30, 50, 60, 100 mg	Q 8, 12, 24 h	Avoid in renal insufficiency
Oxycodone	10, 15, 20, 30, 40, 80 mg	Q 8, 12 h	
Fentanyl transdermal patch	12, 25, 50, 75, 100 mcg/h	Q 48, 72 h	
Methadone	5, 10 mg	Q 6, 8h, 12	Wait 3–5 days between dose increases. Watch for prolonged QT interval and other arrhythmias. Recommended for experienced prescribers only
Oxymorphone	5, 7.5, 10, 15, 20, 30, 40 mg	Q 12 h	

The five commonly used choices of opioids with prolonged effects are depicted in Table 2. All have both pros and cons:

Morphine's metabolite, morphine-3 glucuronide, accumulates with renal insufficiency and may produce toxicity in the form of sedation, confusion, or myoclonus. Many preparations are inexpensive.

Methadone acts as an opioid agonist and an N-methyl d-aspartate (NMDA) antagonist. The latter mechanism may provide advantages in neuropathic pain. Methadone is particularly inexpensive. The pace of titration is more gradual than other strong opioids due to its prolonged terminal half-life but intermediate duration of analgesia. Fatal ventricular arrhythmias have occurred with methadone at high doses (such as greater than 300 mg/day), particularly when prescribed to patients with heart disease and metabolic disarray. Thus methadone prescribing should be reserved for clinicians with experience.

Fentanyl transdermal patches are changed every 72 h or sometimes every 48 h. Febrile patients may have a more rapid and less predictable accumulation of drug in the subcutaneous tissue. For patients requiring very high doses of opioids, it may be impractical to use transdermal fentanyl beyond a few hundred mcg per hour (i.e., three or four 100 mcg/h patches) which is equivalent to the potency of 300–400 mg/day of oxycodone.

Sustained-release tablet formulations of oxycodone, morphine, or oxymorphone tablets must not be cut, crushed, or chewed because that violates the sustained-release structure of the tablets which leads to release of the entire dosage. Sustained-release morphine also comes in capsules containing time-release beads. The beads can be sprinkled on applesauce for ingestion, maintaining the extended release effects.

Ms. N's end-stage renal disease makes morphine a less desirable choice due to potential accumulation of metabolites. Her impulsive behavior and compliance barriers make methadone, which must be titrated with great care, a poor choice. Sustained-release tablets would be a good choice if chewing or breaking is not anticipated. Fentanyl transdermal patches may also reduce impulsive use.

Table 3
Opioid equivalences

Drug	Oral (mg)	IV/SQ (mg except as noted)
Morphine	30	10
Oxycodone	20	–
Hydromorphone	7.5	1.5
Methadone[a]	5	2.5
Fentanyl[b]	–	20 mcg/h IV/TD
Hydrocodone	30	–
Oxymorphone	10	–

Equivalence doses are based on opioid naïve patients

[a]The methadone conversion here is appropriate for moderate doses of opioids. See Walker et al (2008) for a detailed account of this drug's complex dose-related conversions

[b]University of Minnesota Medical Center uses this fentanyl conversion which equates 20 mg of oral oxycodone per day to 20 mcg/h IV infusion or transdermal fentanyl

Opioid starting doses depend on prior opioid exposure. Ms. N has been taking six to eight hydrocodone 5 mg tablets per day which is equal to 30–40 mg hydrocodone per day. To determine the transdermal fentanyl dose that would be equipotent to her daily hydrocodone, refer to the opioid equivalence table (Table 3).

Hydrocodone, 30 mg/day, is equivalent in analgesic potency to 20 mcg/h of transdermal fentanyl. So, hydrocodone, 40 mg/day, would be equivalent to about 27 mcg/h of transdermal fentanyl. When converting from one opioid to another, calculate the equivalent dose but undercut by at least 25–50% to account for incomplete cross tolerance. That is the tolerance that develops after a patient has previously been on one opioid that is not fully transferred to a new opioid exposure. Ms. N will start on a 25 mcg/h fentanyl transdermal patch changed every 72 h. She will continue to use hydrocodone/acetaminophen 5/500 mg up to four per day for breakthrough pain.

To minimize risk with opioid prescribing, increase structure to the prescribing process by having prescriptions renewed weekly or every other week, at least initially. Once satisfactory and predictable dosing is achieved, the frequency of refills can change. This also helps the patient and physician build a relationship and communication. Ms. N's mother might be asked to take on a medication dispensing role, but that may overburden an exhausted caregiver and the mother–daughter relationship.

Ms. N's Case Summary

Pain assessment. Multiregional joint and bone pain due to renal osteodystrophy with fractures and associated muscle dysfunction.

Contributing factors. Weight-bearing and anxiety.

Barriers. Hearing and visual impairment limits communication and increases social isolation. Anger interferes with successful communication and care. Noncompliance negatively affects treatment.

Treatment plan. Begin fentanyl transdermal patch 25 mcg/h every 72 h. Continue up to four hydrocodone/acetaminophen per day, but expect less need. Initiate a trial of a new NSAID and begin calcitonin nasal spray, one spray per day alternating nostrils. Refer to physical therapy for evaluation including possible assistive devices to facilitate increased function and mobility and a TENS trial for additional regional pain management. Follow-up in clinic for prescription refills weekly for the first month and then every 2 weeks.

Things to Tell Ms. N

I want to help you control your pain as much as possible. You have a serious pain problem because of your kidney and bone disease. We will use strong pain medicines – even stronger than your Vicodin; but none of the pain medicines can do this alone. We have to attack the problem from different directions. We can start a fentanyl patch that is as strong as taking about six Vicodin per day. Each patch will last 3 days and will be working even when you are asleep. You may still use up to four Vicodin per day if you need to, but I think you will find that you do not need it so much. When you do take it, it will work better for you. Even though you tried the NSAID before, I think it is a good idea to try another one together with a nasal spray that strengthens your bones and may help bone pain. I want to make sure we get the medicines and other treatments correct and on track, so I am going to ask you to see me every week for a few weeks so we can make adjustments if we need to. I will send you to a physical therapist who will help you find ways to do more with less pain like walking and climbing stairs. She will also let you try a stimulator that you can use when your pain flares up in certain places. Even though there will probably always be some pain, I know there is plenty of room for you to feel better with these and other changes we can make.

SCENARIO 5:
ANOTHER CASE TO APPLY SOME OF THE SAME PRINCIPLES

Mr. P is a 76-year-old man with non-small-cell lung cancer, metastatic to multiple vertebrae and ribs. He has a large tumor mass compressing the right brachial plexus. His pain is described as continual burning and electric shock-like pains occurring with use of his right arm and hand. He has severe aching pain in the mid back. He takes sustained-release morphine 120 mg every 8 h and oxycodone 5 mg every 6 h for breakthrough pain. Pain is rated 8 out of 10 with medication. He is becoming sedated and confused from a dose increase to 120 mg/day, initiated 2 weeks ago. He has not slept in 3 days and has not moved his bowels in 5 days. His family is supportive and ready to help in any way they can to allow him to remain at home until death.

Pain assessment. Cancer-related pain due to spine metastases and tumor invasion of the right brachial plexus. Rule out spinal cord compression. Pain is both bone pain and neuropathic pain. The burden of disease is very high and a palliative approach should be taken.

Contributing factors. Right upper extremity activity, opioid-induced constipation.

Barriers. Opioid-induced central nervous system toxicity at subanalgesic doses.

Treatment plan. Given Mr. P's age, some renal insufficiency is anticipated and thus accumulating morphine metabolites are probably causing sedation and confusion. Switching to a different opioid is likely to reduce these side effects. Methadone would be a good choice since its metabolites do not accumulate with renal insufficiency and the NMDA receptor blocking properties may help reduce his neuropathic pain. *There are numerous conversion charts for methadone, which are dose-dependent and complicated. However, please refer elsewhere for methadone conversions (see Walker et al 2008). In the conversion table above, we based the methadone equivalence on moderate opioid doses. His 360 mg of oral morphine per day is converted, to 60 mg of methadone per day* Accounting for incomplete cross tolerance, it is prescribed as *15 mg every 8 h.* Initiating a bowel regimen is key when starting opioids. This should include a laxative with or without a stool softener. (For more on constipation, please see Chap. 7.)

Adding an adjuvant may enhance the effects on neuropathic pain. Choices include anticonvulsants, tricyclic antidepressants, dexamethasone, and others. Tricyclic antidepressants have the potential for intolerable side effects in the elderly: orthostatic hypotension, sedation, cardiac arrhythmias, and anticholinergic effects. Anticonvulsants are effective for neuropathic pain and have little or no drug–drug interactions. Their toxicity is relatively low and primarily related to sedation that is dose-dependent. Dexamethasone can dramatically reduce neuropathic pain due to tumor invasion or compression of nerves as well as tumor-related edema. Dexamethasone also has a robust impact on bone pain due to metastases and Mr. P may have a spinal cord compression from epidural invasion of one or more of his thoracic vertebral metastases. This would also warrant the use of dexamethasone both for pain control and for improvement in neurologic function.

Mr. P's pain improves over the next 48 h. He is more alert and coherent. Pain is still rated at 7 out of 10. He is asking if the methadone can be increased. How can the pain medication be titrated up to achieve optimal pain control?

Among the opioids, methadone is the most difficult to titrate because of its long terminal half-life. Tissue saturation and plasma redistribution occur after about 3–5 days so with repeated dosing there can be increased analgesia and also increased sedation after a few days. Therefore, with methadone, dose adjustments should be made cautiously and at intervals of no less than 3–5 days. Meanwhile, using analgesics for breakthrough pain that are shorter acting and that have simpler kinetics provides the bridge for interval time between methadone titrations. The dose of breakthrough opioid should be proportional to the total daily dose of opioid – 5–15% of the daily dose. Mr. P's total daily of 45 mg oral methadone is equivalent to 180 mg/day of oxycodone. Ten percent of 180 mg is about 20 mg of oxycodone. That would be an appropriate breakthrough dose of oxycodone for Mr. P to take every 3–4 h. If we monitor his use of oxycodone for breakthrough pain, then we can calculate how much to increase his methadone after about 5 days. If Mr. P takes an average four doses or 80 mg of oxycodone per day in the previous 5 days, we can increase the daily methadone accordingly. 80 mg of oxycodone is equivalent to 20 mg of methadone; so we will increase Mr. P's methadone from 45 to 65 mg/day or a little less. We will adjust Mr. P's dose to 20 mg every 8 h and continue the oxycodone at 20 mg or perhaps 25 mg every 3–4 h.

After several months of stable pain control, Mr. P develops a new headache with an increase in back and neck pain. Cerebral metastases are found and bone metastases are widespread throughout the entire spine, multiple ribs, and long bones. Mr. P is hospitalized for pain control in the terminal phases of his disease. His family is pleading to do whatever it takes to keep him comfortable. He is able to tell you that pain is severe and he wants comfort measures only. What should be done with the opioid analgesics?

Parenteral opioids allow for aggressive titration to comfort and the avoidance of the GI tract in this sedated patient.

To start a hydromorphone infusion:

- Discontinue the methadone.
- Begin an infusion equivalent to the total daily dose of methadone, 60 mg, plus oxycodone, about 100 mg.
- If 1.5 mg of IV hydromorphone is equivalent to 5 mg of oral methadone (Table 3), the total daily home doses thus equal about 18 mg + 7.5 mg, or about 25 mg/day of IV hydro-

Table 4

Sample 24 h titration of hydromorphone infusion every 4 h based on incorporating PRN doses given in a 4 h interval

Hour	1	2	3	4	5	6	7	8	9	10	11	12	13	14	15	16	17	18	19	20	21	22	23	24
PRN mg	4	6	4	4	3	2	2	4	4	6	4	0	0	6	4	3	3	2	3	3	2	0	0	2
Infusion rate mg/h	1	1	1	1	5	5	5	5	7	7	7	7	10	10	10	10	13	13	13	13	15	15	15	15

Each new infusion rate represents the average hourly use of PRN doses of hydromorphone rounded down morphone. The basis of this calculation is that 60 mg of oral methadone is equivalent to 18 mg of IV hydromorphone and 100 mg of oral oxycodone is equivalent to 7.5 mg of IV hydromorphone.

- Therefore, start a hydromorphone infusion at 1 mg/h. We will do a straight conversion without downsizing for cross tolerance due to the acute analgesic needs at this terminal state where avoiding sedation has less priority. *Outside the terminal state, providing about 50–60% of the calculated dose as a continuous infusion with breakthrough pain dosing allows for careful assessment and helps achieve the best results.*
- Nursing staff should assess pain and response to medicine every 30–60 min at first, and give additional IV/SQ hydromorphone as indicated.

  – Pain assessment can take the form of patient report, if possible, and observation of pain behaviors (e.g., moaning, grimacing, extremity withdrawal, or guarding movements).

  – When pain has improved and is stable, assessments may be spaced out every 2 h. The opioid infusion should be adjusted every 4 h according to how much nurse-administered hydromorphone had to be added in the previous 4 h. Using this titration process, the opioid doses can, if necessary, climb rapidly over just 24 h as depicted in Table 4.

If excessive side effects occur, the continuous infusion can be reduced to the rate used in the previous 4 h. If there is adequate pain control but excessive sedation and a central nervous system stimulant is indicated, try methylphenidate 5–10 mg, dextroamphetamine 5–30 mg, or modafinil 100–200 mg given in the morning.

The two cases presented in this chapter illustrate the wide spectrum of pain in the palliative care setting. This spectrum is emphasized on a continuum of disease burden that includes both early on and end-of-life pain. The goals and approach to pain management are largely determined by where a patient is on this disease burden spectrum. Using treatments specific for the cardinal pain types – nociceptive, neuropathic, muscle, and bone – is crucial. Identifying and addressing contributing factors and barriers frequently represent the missing links in unsuccessful pain treatment regimens. Opioids and opioid titration play a key role in more advanced illness. Knowing the relative potencies of the different opioids and of the various routes of administration allows the clinician to tailor the medication to the needs of the patient.

FURTHER READING

Chen H, Lamer TJ, Rho RH et al (2004) Contemporary management of neuropathic pain for the primary care physician. Mayo Clin Proc 79(12):1533–1545

Fine PG, Low, CM (2006) Principles of effective pain management at the end of life. MedScape from WebMD, 5 Oct 2006. http://www.medscape.com/viewarticle/545562

Halvorson KG, Sevick MA, Ghilardi JR et al (2006) Similarities and differences in tumor growth, skeletal remodeling and pain in an osteolytic and osteoblastic model of bone cancer. Clin J Pain Sep 22(6):587–600

Mantyh PW, Clohisy DR, Koltzenburg M, Hunt SP (2002) Molecular mechanisms of cancer pain. Nat Rev Cancer 2:201–209

McNicol E (2007) Opioid side effects: pain clinical updates. Int Assoc Study Pain XV(2):1–6

Walker P, Palla S, Pei B et al (2008) Switching from methadone to a different opioid: what is the equi-analgesic dose ratio. J Palliative Med 11(8):1103–1108

9

Palliative Wound and Skin Issues

Cynthia A. Worley

ABSTRACT

Normal wound healing follows specific, predictable patterns. Systemic and local factors such as chronic illness and cancer treatment can affect the patient's ability to heal. The goals of treatment must therefore reflect the patient's current medical condition and ability to heal. Appropriate skin care measure must be taken for the patient with end-stage disease. Often palliative care patients will not be able to heal their wounds. It is important to remember that the clinician cannot "make a patient's wounds heal," but must support the patient, their family, and symptoms until death.

Key Words: Wound healing; Skin care; Skin repair process; Heal; Palliative care

CONSIDER

1. The effect of chronic illness on wound healing
2. The effect of cancer treatment on wound healing
3. Inability of marshaling an appropriate wound healing response
4. Appropriate skin care measures for the patient with end-stage disease

KEY POINTS

- Normal wound healing follows specific, predictable patterns.
- Systemic and local factors contribute to the patient's ability to heal.
- Chronic illness impacts the normal skin repair process.
- The goals of treatment must reflect the patient's current medical condition and ability to heal.
- Often palliative care patients will not be able to heal their wounds.

From: *Current Clinical Oncology: Palliative Care: A Case-based Guide,*
Edited by: J.E. Loitman et al. DOI: 10.1007/978-1-60761-590-3_9,
© Springer Science+Business Media, LLC 2010

- The clinician cannot "make a patient's wound heal."
- The clinician can only establish or attempt to establish and support an optimal moist wound healing environment.

SCENARIO 1:
COMPREHENSIVE ASSESSMENT

Ms. L is a 50-year-old patient diagnosed and treated for breast cancer. She is treated with chemotherapy followed by radiation and surgery for disease that had metastasized to her liver, bone, and lung. She has developed radiation necrosis following completion of that treatment.

Establishing good wound care is based on the foundation of an accurate assessment and a treatment plan that meets the goals of the patient. The job of the palliative care clinician is to ensure the right environment to allow a patient's body to heal the wound or at least not allow the wound to deteriorate if possible. Wound healing with any chronic advanced illness is the complex balance of many different arenas for the patient. In palliative care patients, this complex balance is further complicated by decreasing functional status and an accumulation of previous injuries, illnesses and side effects from past treatments.

Normal Wound Healing

The normal process of wound healing consists of three phases: inflammation, proliferation, and maturation. These phases are not discrete and isolated but overlap, ebb, and flow depending upon the patient's current medical condition.

During inflammation, the goal is to reestablish a protective barrier to prevent bacterial invasion and restore hemostasis. This phase should also facilitate elimination of foreign material and devitalized tissue through a natural debridement process. Once the inflammatory phase is resolving, various cells involved in the regeneration or repair of tissue "proliferate" in the patient's wound and begin the process of filling the defect with connective tissue (granulation) or regenerating exact replicas of damaged tissue. Wound dimensions decrease in size in larger, deeper wounds, also referred to as wound contracture. Resurfacing follows with new epithelial cells at the wound edge beginning to cover the more superficial wound bed. When the wound surface is completely restored, the wound bed matures through strengthening the collagen matrix (in full-thickness or deeper wounds). Over time, the area develops increased wound tensile strength which improves the patient's ability to resist external mechanical forces. However, the ultimate tensile strength achieved is often weaker than intact skin.

Principles of wound healing

- Identify etiology of wound
- Remove necrotic tissue and control infection/"bioburden"
- Support normal wound healing
- Create optimal environment for healing

Factors Effecting Wound Healing

A goal of healing aims for restoration of structure and function to the skin after tissue damage. In an optimal environment and with enough time, all wounds would heal adequately. However, there are many roadblocks to optimal wound healing.

Roadblock to healing	Role of interference
Inadequate nutrition	Malnutrition decreases visceral proteins which are key in all phases of healing especially proliferation of granulation tissue and new blood vessel generation
Poor tissue perfusion and oxygenation	Hypoxia impairs granulation tissue formation and phagocytic activity
Comorbidities	Diabetes alters immune responses; Cardiac and respiratory diseases interfere with perfusion and oxygenation; Malignancies exhaust nutritional stores. Consider the impacted physiology of any systemic illness
Medications	"Statin" drugs may interfere with new blood vessel generation; Steroids inhibit normal inflammation and wound repair; Antineoplastic agents (chemotherapy) interfere with all rapidly proliferating cells
Necrotic tissue	Harbors bacteria
Bacterial contamination/infection	Competes with normal healthy cells for nutrients and oxygen; bacteria produce toxins which harm healthy tissue
Cancer treatment	Radiation alters normal wound healing in the radiation field; chemotherapy delays wound healing by suppressing proliferation of cells involved in wound healing
Poor functional status	Bedbound or poorly mobile patients without support cannot relieve pressure to allow wounds to heal

Other systemic factors such as stress, body build, and age will also contribute to challenges to wound healing. It is important to have a thorough knowledge of the patient's treatment history and current status prior to determining treatment goals and developing an appropriate plan of care.

SCENARIO 2:
TREATMENT GOALS

A year later, Ms. L is found to have a necrotic tumor in the right chest wall which is surgically resected. She develops a nonhealing wound in the previously irradiated field. She is subsequently placed on maintenance therapy using Tamoxifen for stable disease. Ms. L has home care for wound monitoring. Despite numerous interventions, Ms. L eventually requires two reconstructive procedures to close the wound.

The treatment plan for any patient with a wound is influenced by the established goals of care, the potential outcomes of treatment, education of the patient and/or family, the use of appropriate materials, and the adherence to the plan of care. Wound management therapies should be included with the overall treatment plan for the patient's disease. Minimizing wound complications to support disease modifying treatments may be a priority. Ms. L is still undergoing active treatment for metastatic breast cancer and her goal is to receive the most potent anticancer agents and to have reconstructive surgery in the future. Patients with illnesses such as chronic obstructive pulmonary disease whose dyspnea severely limits their mobility, the risk for pressure ulcer development is increased. In patients with a connective tissue disease, such as Lupus Erythematosus or Scleroderma, whose disease affects their epidermis, wound healing may be poor. Prevention and minimization of complications are other goals that patients will prioritize.

Patients with poorly healing wounds often become very frustrated at the apparent lack of progress toward healing. Radiation therapy permanently alters the patient's healing ability in the irradiated area. Surgical incisions in previous radiation sites frequently fail to close properly and the resulting wound consists of tissue which is inelastic and inflexible, unable to withstand mechanical forces and poorly vascularized. The need for psychosocial or psychiatric support should be assessed with regards to wound healing and body image.

SCENARIO 3:
DISEASE PROGRESSION AND MOBILITY

> *After 2 years of medical quiescence, Ms. L is admitted for respiratory failure secondary to possible aspiration pneumonia related to vomiting. She is now bed bound and having diarrhea from the enteral nutrition.*

The prevention of skin breakdown rests on identification of risk factors. As patients' diseases progress, their inherent risk increases from multiple areas. Risk factors include measuring the patient's activity, mobility, nutritional status, risk for incontinence, mental status, and risk of skin damage from friction and shear. Patients may experience decreased appetite with subsequent decrease in nutritionally significant intake which may affect healing. They may also become less active from weakness, pain, loss of functional mobility, or problems with perfusion and oxygenation. When patients become bed- or chair-fast, for whatever reason, their risk for potential skin breakdown increases. Patients who sleep in a recliner at home because of severe pulmonary disease or who are bed bound and unable to turn are significantly at risk for skin breakdown in the heel, sacral, gluteal, and coccygeal areas. Ms. L is at risk for wounds in the sacral, thoracic, and heel areas because of her immobility, poor nutritional status, and decreased activity levels.

In 2009, the Joint Commission made "healthcare associated pressure ulcers" a National Patient Safety Goal. This decision was spurred by the incidence of hospital-acquired pressure ulcers and the associated costs of treatment. As the Centers for Medicare Services will no longer reimburse hospitals for the costs associated with treatment of hospital-acquired pressure ulcers, the Joint Commission has made pressure ulcer risk identification and prevention a priority in all healthcare settings.

Use of a risk assessment tool such as the Braden Scale is recommended and seen in many healthcare facilities. Risk assessments should be performed by nursing staff on all patients upon admission to any facility, routinely during admission and whenever there is a change in the patient's condition. The Braden Scale is a tool used to predict risk for the development of pressure ulcers. Below are potential responses to particular risk factors. These can be found at www.bradenscale.com.

Risk factors	Actions to consider ...
Decreased activity	Physical or occupational therapy to increase or improve strength for ADLs
	Assess medications to decrease limitations
Decreased mobility	Consider increasing turning schedule
	Use of specialized mattresses
	Use of lift sheets or mechanical assistive devices for repositioning
Impaired nutritional status	Strategies to improve or increase appetite
	Favorite foods
	Small frequent meals
	Treat dry mouth
Incontinence	Apply moisture barriers ointments
	Emollient cleansers to maintain normal skin pH
	Eliminate use of briefs which hold urine and stool close to the skin
	Consider bladder catheter/rectal tube rectal pouch if stools are frequent
Friction and shear	Frequent use of positioning devices
	Raise the foot of the bed to prevent patient sliding across bed linens
Altered mental status	Judicious use of restraints with careful monitoring of the patient
	Calm peaceful environment

Pressure Ulcers

The National Pressure Ulcer Advisory Panel (NPUAP) defines a pressure ulcer as "an area of localized injury to the skin and/or underlying tissue, usually over a bony prominence, which results from pressure or pressure in combination with friction and/or shear." The staging system developed by this panel of experts has been the "gold standard" used to determine level of tissue injury worldwide. To ensure consistent description of wounds, many facilities choose to have ready access to laminated charts with pictures and descriptions of the various stages.

Stage	Description
I	Intact skin
	Nonblanchable redness of a localized area
	Usually over a bony prominence
	May be difficult to detect in individuals with darker skin tones
II	Partial-thickness tissue loss
	Shallow open ulcer with a red/pink wound bed
	May be shiny or dry in appearance
	No slough
	May also present as an intact or open/ruptured serum-filled blister
III	Full thickness tissue loss
	Subcutaneous fat may be visible
	Bone, tendon, or muscle not exposed
	+/− Slough
	+/− Undermining and/or tunneling

(continued)

(continued)

Stage	Description
IV	Full thickness tissue loss
	Exposed bone, tendon or muscle
	+/– Slough
	+/– Partial Eschar
	Often include undermining and tunneling
Unstageable	Full thickness tissue loss
	Full covereage by:
	Slough (yellow, tan, gray, green, or brown)
	and/or
	Eschar (tan, brown, or black)
Suspected deep tissue injury	Intact skin
	Purple or maroon localized area
	or
	Blood-filled blister due to damage of underlying soft tissue

Two months later, Ms. L is admitted to the Intensive Care Unit following cardiac arrest. She is ventilator-dependent and receives a tracheostomy. She has multiple areas of skin breakdown along the thoracic spine due to curvature. Her goal of care continues to be disease treatment aimed at cure. A change in the nutritional formula fails to reduce her stool frequency. At this point, she experiences skin erosion from frequent stools.

The choice of skin barrier product is dictated by the cause of the skin irritation. If the patient is incontinent of urine or stool, frequent changing of pads or diapers is warranted to prevent breakdown. The use of any device which allows urine or stool to remain in constant contact with the skin should be discouraged. Bladder or rectal catheters divert urine and stool away from the skin.

The choice of wound dressing should be dictated by the wound characteristics and the treatment needs. There are many different types of wound dressings available.

While gauze dressings may appear to be the simplest, most easily applied type of dressing, there are many advanced wound care products which may be the "better choice" for wound care. Below is not an inclusive list, but will provide some basic information about different types of dressings available.

Dressing type	Description	Possible uses
Transparent films	Usually polyurethane membranes coated with an adhesive which will not stick to the wound bed. Unable to absorb drainage but can protect superficial wounds	Skin tears – reapproximate wound edges prior to application. Friction injury. Ruptured blisters or bullae – use caution when removing
Hydrocolloids	Hydrophyllic particles which are bound within a matrix. Outer layer is usually a thin film or polyurethane foam. Absorb drainage by particle swelling	Use on wounds with small to moderate amounts of drainage – partial-thickness pressure ulcers, venous leg ulcers, or arterial ulcers. Exercise caution when removing as adhesives are strong

(continued)

(continued)

Dressing type	Description	Possible uses
Hydrogels	Predominantly water-based, dressings are either amorphous (gel form) or bound in an inert matrix (sheet form). Not particularly absorbent due to high water content	Provide soothing and cooling benefit May be used on partial-thickness wounds, wounds from ionizing radiation, itching
Foams	Usually made from polyurethane polymers which are hydrophilic and absorptive. Available in adhesive and nonadhesive forms	Use on small to moderately draining wounds, depending upon thickness, Pressure ulcers Skin tears Traumatic injuries Lower extremity ulcers
Alginates	Derived from seaweed fibers, these dressings are capable of managing larger amounts of drainage	Use on wounds with moderate to heavy drainage. Requires secondary dressing
Composite dressings	These dressings are "combination" products made from two or more materials which are physically distinct but manufactured together	Use as cover dressings to assist with drainage management or as single dressings over tube sites or IV lines. The amount of wound exudate will determine the appropriate composite dressing
Contact layers	These dressings are designed to prevent adhesion of dressing materials to the wound bed. May be woven or nonwoven	Use for packing painful wounds
Antimicrobial dressings	Available in both pad and gel form, these dressings are designed to control bacteria present in wounds – may contain substances such as cadexomer iodine, silver, or polyhexamethylene	Use on wounds with significant colonization or bioburden and are often used in combination with other dressings

SCENARIO 4:
FOCUSED SYMPTOM MANAGEMENT

Ms. L is now nonresponsive. Her wounds and medical condition have deteriorated. Her family believes that she will be cured. They do accept help from the Palliative Care Team and an increased focus on symptom management. There is some odor associated with the thoracic wounds. Some family members avoid visiting due to the bad odor in Ms. L's room. They are also concerned that the systemic pain medicine is sedating her so much that she cannot wake up to interact with them.

While patients are concerned about their wounds, there are certain wound characteristics about which will significantly increase a patient's anxiety about dressings and dressing changes. As mentioned previously, some types of wounds will cause such problems as to alter the patient's lifestyle, cause them to become isolated or avoid family and friends. In these instances, certain care strategies may assist in allowing them to continue their normal activities.

Possible patient concern	Treatment goal	Dressing or treatment option
Odor management	Control or minimize the wound "smell"	• Use of charcoal dressing – activated charcoal layers in certain dressings will filter air molecules • Use of dilute antiseptic solution – necrotic tissues, tumors, and devitalized tissues harbor odor-causing bacteria – may try dilute acetic acid solution, ¼ strength Daikins (0.125% buffered Clorox ™ – do not use any other type of bleach) – limit use of these solutions to 7–10 days
Pain management	Minimize patient pain and discomfort during dressing changes	• Systemic premedication with opioids analgesics, allowing 30 min for oral or 10 min for parenteral doses • Routinely administer NSAIDs for the inflammatory component • Apply topical anesthetics such as 2% Xylocaine, EMLA cream™, or 4% topical Lidocaine solution • Apply topical morphine 0.125% in thin layer
Drainage management	Minimize frequency of dressing changes, minimize potential for maceration and tissue trauma from dressing removal	• Use absorptive dressings such as alginates and hydrofibers • Use absorbent secondary dressings • "Pouching system" such as a drainage ostomy pouch or wound manager • Drainage management system such as negative pressure wound therapy

Many patients with large, malodorous, or unsightly wounds will either isolate themselves or become isolated because of the wound symptoms. In addition to the dressings listed above, placing odor absorbing material under the bed can reduce the immediate room odor. Such materials could be a bowl of baking soda, charcoal, kitty litter, or coffee grounds. Ventilating the room depends on the patient's tolerance.

Additional applications for wound odor include metronidazole powder, crushed metronidazole tablets, topical antibiotic solutions, or dilute antiseptic solutions to reduce bacterial burden and thus gaseous odors.

Some treatments for wound pain include using medications in an off-label manner. This is difficult, if not impossible, in hospitals and intensive care units but may be possible in nursing facilities, in hospice and palliative care units, and in home hospice. The application of morphine with or without viscous lidocaine to open wounds can reduce pain and systemic opioid needs.

Being prepared for the risk of bleeding is essential. Elimination of NSAIDS and anticoagulants needs consideration. Have alginates or silver nitrate sticks available for hemostasis or absorption of small areas. For severe bleeding, make dark towels available to absorb the blood and reduce the impact on caregivers and loved ones.

Sometimes, despite our best efforts to prevent skin breakdown, patients are incapable of maintaining their skin integrity and the skin begins to fail. As patients' medical condition deteriorates, their risk for breakdown increases. The patient may develop an area on a dependent, bony prominence which takes on a "bruised" appearance; the skin becomes purple or maroon in color. There is no obvious breakdown but the discoloration is present and will ultimately lead to an opening in the skin if pressure remains constant. Fecal and urinary incontinence can contribute to skin breakdown due to the excessive moisture levels and presence of digestive enzymes in the stool. Appropriate use of skin barriers is necessary for patient comfort and to preserve intact skin. The normal routine of pressure relief by turning or the use of specialty beds may not be appropriate for the imminently dying patient.

FURTHER READING

de la Torre JI, Tobin GR (1998) Physiology and healing dynamics of chronic cutaneous wounds. Am J Surg 176(2A Suppl):26S–38S

Fonder M, Lazarua G, Cowan D, Aronson-Cook B, Kohli A, Mamelak A (2008) Treating the chronic wound: a practical approach to the care of nonhealing wounds and wound care dressings. J Am Acad Dermatol 58:185–206

Lyder CH, Presto J, Grady J, Scinto J, Allman R, Bergstrom N et al (2001) Quality of care for hospitalized medicare patients at risk for pressure ulcers. Arch Intern Med 161(12):1549–1554

Niezgoda JA, Mendez-Eastman S (2005) Effective management of pressure ulcers. Adv Skin Wound Care 19(Suppl 1):3–15

Worley CA (2005) So, what do I put on this wound? Making sense of the wound dressing puzzle: Part I, II, and III. Dermatol Nurs 17:143–144, 204–105, 299–300

Wound Ostomy and Continence Nurses Society (2003) Guideline for prevention and management of pressure ulcers. Wound Ostomy and Continence Nurses Society, Glenview, IL

10 Issues in the Last Hours

Jane E. Loitman and Christian T. Sinclair

ABSTRACT

The foundation of good end-of-life care involves assessment, education, treatment, and reassessment. Effective symptom management and attention to the quality of life for patients and families are the primary goals of palliative care. This care often shifts to the needs of the family such that communication and education about the dying process, the medications, and the unspoken questions become a priority. Grief may be present before death and should be addressed by the team when observed. Evaluation of grief should include inquiry about after-death religious traditions and preparation for signing of the death certificate.

Key Words: Assessment; Symptom management; Palliative care; Burial; Education; Death; End-of-life care; Double effect; Euthanasia; Physician-assisted suicide

> *Mrs. D is a 79-year-old mother of five with a long history of Chronic Obstructive Pulmonary Disease and Coronary Artery Disease. She is admitted for worsening dyspnea and concurrent anxiety related to her difficulty breathing. Three days later, she is resting comfortably, but is minimally responsive with her immediate family at her bedside around the clock.*

CONSIDER

1. What if her family felt treating her symptoms hastened death?
2. What if her dyspnea had not resolved?
3. What specifics must one remember once Mrs. D expired?

From: *Current Clinical Oncology: Palliative Care: A Case-based Guide,*
Edited by: J.E. Loitman et al. DOI: 10.1007/978-1-60761-590-3_10,
© Springer Science + Business Media, LLC 2010

KEY POINTS

- The foundation of good end-of-life care is to: assess, educate, treat, and reassess.
- Effective symptom management and attention to the quality of life for patients and families are the primary goals of palliative care.
- Symptom management for pain, dyspnea, and other common symptoms does not hasten death.
- Double effect is an ethical construct relating to aggressive symptom management with an understanding that death may be an unintended consequence.
- Euthanasia is the act and intent of hastening of death by medications administered by a health care professional.
- Physician-assisted suicide is the act and intent of hastening death by medications administered by the patient with the endorsement of the physician.
- Care often shifts to the needs of the family in the last few days as education about the dying process and medications becomes a priority.
- Inquire about after-death religious traditions.
- Grief may be present before death and should be addressed by the team when observed.
- Familiarize yourself with regional requirements regarding death certificates and impact on timing of burial and cremation.

SCENARIO 1:
EFFECTIVE TREATMENT OF SYMPTOMS IN THE LAST DAYS OF LIFE

Mrs. D is extremely short of breath causing her to appear very anxious as she looks rapidly around the room and moves from sitting to standing and back to sitting. Dyspnea limits her subjective assessment, but her daughter is helpful in mentioning that these "episodes" happen three to five times every day and seem to get better once she takes her lorazepam and morphine. "The nebulizers don't always seem to help. Sometimes they make her claustrophobic," adds her daughter. Mrs. D whispers with much effort, "I just don't .... want ... me ... suffocate."

Foundation of good end-of-life care and symptom management

- Assess
- Educate
- Treat
- Reassess

   In the last few days and hours of life, patients are unlikely able to give a detailed report of their symptoms secondary to decreasing cognition as a result of the disease burden, the dying process and possibly medications. In assessing a minimally responsive patient, take great care to observe any nonverbal signs of distress, such as frowning, tense body posture, moaning, and other appearance of discomfort. Ask family members and other staff about their observances of any unease the patient has demonstrated. All together this may give a more accurate picture of symptom severity.

Assess

Nonverbal signs of distress
Team assessment of patient
Severity of symptoms

Related symptoms
Effectiveness of past therapies
Ineffectiveness of past therapies
Tolerance to medications
Goal of symptom control

Understanding the history of symptoms and past effectiveness of therapies to control symptoms is essential for a good assessment of symptoms. Occasionally, inquiring specifically about therapies with a significant degree of ineffectiveness avoids increased time of continuing poor symptom control. Tolerance to medication, particularly opioids and benzodiazepines, will guide titration in addition to severity of symptoms. Asking the patient or family about the goals of symptom control assists the clinician in determining the frequency of assessments and medication adjustments required to meet the goals. Mrs. D is afraid of suffocation indicating nonpharmacologic care may also be helpful.

You discuss with the daughter and patient the plan to continue her current doses of oxycodone and lorazepam and make nebulizers available as needed. In anticipation of needing more opioids for her dyspnea, you also discuss the possibility of using long-acting opioids, and confide a desire to continue to work together to avoid the feeling of suffocation. You also caution them about somnolence and constipation with more aggressive medication administration.

Comprehensive education about the treatment plan and expected outcomes reduces patient and family anxiety. Reviewing both pharmacologic and nonpharmacologic measures for symptom management and quality of life care avoids potential errors and false assumptions. Discussing expected side effects or changes to the patients' functional or cognitive status enhances the family's understanding of the dying process.

As the hospice/palliative care team works together in treating the patient and supporting the family, reassessment of symptoms and concerns becomes an important role for excellent whole patient care. Evaluating the amount and effectiveness of medications to control symptoms guides the educational focus for the patient and family.

Education

Know indications and limitations of medications
Discuss expectations of disease course with regard to symptoms and death
Consider and discuss continuing or discontinuing medications no longer helpful
Chronic medications for example iron and cholesterol
Symptom medications for example stimulants
Advise caregivers – family to assume the patient who is no longer conscious can still hear
Discuss issues related to IV fluids and the diminished value of nutrition

Opioids can cause respiratory depression although this is a rare phenomenon in patients who are tolerant, have ongoing pain, and are taking opioids judiciously for symptom management. For that reason, it is imperative that health care providers who care for patients at the end of life become familiar and comfortable with prescribing and utilizing opioids for their patients.

For more details on opioids, please refer to Chap. ? on Pulmonary Symptoms and Chap. ? on Opioids for Pain Control.

The next morning you see Mrs. D and she appears more comfortable. She arouses to say a few words without being short of breath. The night nurse reports Mrs. D had her respiratory rate decrease to 8 overnight with occasional apneic episodes lasting 10 s. She received multiple doses of opioids and benzodiazepines.

Opioids are a powerful tool in treating both pain and dyspnea. The general public and healthcare professionals fear this class of medications for their association with addiction and respiratory suppression. Palliative care clinicians can confidently educate patients and families, dutifully administer them when indicated, and avoid undue harm to the patient by understanding opioid pharmacology. In the last few hours to days of life, medicating symptoms becomes an art based on science because side effects of medication can be difficult to differentiate from the dying process.

Families and patients may request a decrease in medications to see if the patient "wakes up" or "has less apnea." Such requests must be balanced by the degree of symptom control that currently exists and the goal of care. If one believes medications are impacting cognition, breathing, or some other aspect, a trial of decreasing the medications may be warranted. When the medications are decreased, it is wise to discuss the plan if dyspnea, pain, or other symptoms return.

Treatment

Specific indications and limitations of pharmacologic symptom management
i.e., management of sialorrhea, dyspnea, delirium, drying of mucous membranes, etc.
Refractory symptom management using polypharmacy
i.e., opioids, neuroleptics, benzodiazepines, anesthetic agents

Sialorrhea and the excessive secretions at the end of life

Both conditions are disturbing to the family and caregivers and deserve treatment.
Secretions pool in the posterior pharynx and the patient is either too weak or not alert enough to clear the secretions. Finding alternate routes for sublingual medications may avoid external contributions to the secretions. Anticholinergics can be of limited use to prevent further secretions:

- Atropine drops (~6) can be placed under the tongue for ease of administration every 2 h
- For patients with weeks to live, scopolamine patches reduce patient–caregiver burden, though it takes 24 h to reach steady state and scopolamine crosses the blood brain barrier which can cause or exacerbate a delirium
- Hyoscyamine sulfate is easy to administer sublingually 0.125 mg every 2–4 h

SCENARIO 2:
RESPIRATORY SUPPRESSION AND HASTENED DEATH

> *Mrs. D's dyspnea worsens. She is able to whisper that opioid gives her the most relief. The nurse receives an order to increase the opioid dose by 10% and then 20%. She stops breathing 20 min after the second opioid dose. A daughter-in-law expresses concern that oxycodone "is killing her, because I heard it could stop your breathing. Is that what you are trying to do here?"*

Unfortunately, aggressive palliative care is often misinterpreted as hastening death. When aggressive symptom management calls for rapid titration of opioids, respiratory depression can occur. The underlying disease process and the dying process also contribute to respiratory depression and it becomes impossible to attribute a one cause. In cases where the goal of care is congruent with relief of symptoms, the doctrine of double effect explains that an act can have both desirable (symptom relief) and undesirable (death) consequences. The act of titrating opioids for Mrs. D's dyspnea caused an effect one would normally be obliged to avoid, Mrs. D's death. While it is permissible to responsibly titrate the opioid for comfort, it is essential to document that the treatment plan is relief of dyspnea and to continue reassess and educate the patient and family. Documentation of failure to control a symptom at current doses is important to justify increasing the dose or changing to a different medication.

SCENARIO 3:
RESPONDING TO A REQUEST FOR HASTENED DEATH

> *That afternoon, a son arrives from out of town and asks to speak with you about his mother's condition. He says, "Mom would never want to lay in bed like this. She is suffering just laying there. Like a vegetable. How long are we going to let this go on? Can't you do something about this?"*

Dealing with requests for hastened death is a challenge for many professionals in hospice and palliative care. Since euthanasia and physician-assisted suicide are illegal in majority of the USA (physician-assisted suicide was legalized in Oregon in 1997), committing these acts could result in criminal charges and loss of professional licensure.

Euthanasia, in contrast to the double effect, is the act and intent of hastening death by medications administered by a health care professional. Physician-assisted suicide is the act and intent of hastening death by medications administered by the patient with the endorsement of the physician.

Elicit more information in response to requests for hastened death. For example, ask why the son feels his mother is suffering, when she appears peaceful and comfortable. Openly discussing expected prognosis can diminish feelings that the current situation is going to persist longer than the family expects. One's desire to work within professional norms to alleviate suffering remains primary though, occasionally, reference to the illegal nature of the act may be relevant. It can be common for families to have disparate views about hastened death including feelings that the hospice or palliative care team desires hastened death. These difficult situations require excellent communication within the interdisciplinary team and with the patient and family.

Be mindful to identify more subtle requests for hastened death. A sarcastic reference to euthanasia may be placed to judge one's response. It is important to educate what is and is not within our control so misperception of secretive hastened death is avoided.

SCENARIO 4:
UNCONTROLLED DYSPNEA AND PALLIATIVE SEDATION

In spite of aggressive titration of medications and implementation of behavioral and environmental techniques, Mrs. D continues to gasp for air and cry that she is suffocating. The son in Scenario 3 arrives but says, "Mom would never want to die like this. She is suffering. Can't you do something to make her unconscious?"

Palliative sedation in the terminal phase of life is a procedure with many different names in the medical literature including "terminal sedation." It is considered an acceptable option in cases where physical suffering persists despite aggressive symptom strategies. More controversy exists over the use of palliative sedation in those who are not imminently dying or who are suffering for psychological or existential reasons. Palliative specialists should be involved in cases utilizing palliative sedation. A consensus with the healthcare providers, the patient, and the family must occur first and documentation is essential. Prior to initiating palliative sedation, the team, family, and patient should discuss code status and the provision or withholding of artificial nutrition.

Palliative sedation medications

Schedule sedating medication and titrate to effect
Multiple sedating medications may be necessary
Continue opioids and titrate accordingly
Opioids alone do not provide sufficient sedation
Utilize sedation with benzodiazepines, neuroleptics, barbiturates, and/or other sedatives
Subcutaneous or intravenous routes are often preferred

SCENARIO 5:
TIME OF DEATH

Mrs. D becomes sedated and comfortable using the strategies of a thorough assessment, education of the patient and family as well as pharmacologic and nonpharmacologic strategies. Her family is gathered around her reflecting on past experiences, as if she could hear. Quietly and subtly, Mrs. D stops breathing.

When patients are enrolled in hospice, families are told to notify the hospice nurse at the time of death if no hospice staff is present. Typically, the nurse goes to the home to pronounce the death and subsequently notifies the funeral home and anyone else who may be desired, such as a chaplain or someone from the patient's religious community. Some religions have specific rituals regarding the body after death so inquiring and helping to implement any traditions is encouraged.

At the time of death, family members will all show grief and sadness in their own manner. Hospice and palliative care staff are encouraged to be open and receptive to these emotions without being overly prescriptive in response. Being present and available to listen are important roles of the medical professional at the time of death. Clichés may be much less effective than silence at times like these.

Pronouncement of death requires the observation of lack of spontaneous heart rate and respiratory rate for at least 1 min. Examinations of the eyes, testing of reflexes, or assessment of the response to pain are not required for an expected death and may be considered disrespectful to the body.

With regard to coroners, autopsies, and death certificates, criteria are enforced locally and may vary. For clinicians with many anticipated deaths or who refer regularly to hospice, understanding local and regional nuances is advised.

When patients are not enrolled in hospice, the same applies though the funeral and death planning and the availability of the hospice nurse will be missing. Additionally, the body will more often be referred to the coroner. Hospice agencies and hospital spiritual care departments are good resources for education.

Death certificates are important sources for data and should be approached with detail and accuracy. The final cause of death and any significant preceding events contributing to the cause of death are areas left for the physician to complete. While many patients do not have such a neat, linear and ordered health history, this information is compiled to track health trends of your community so the most complete information is preferred, including histology of cancers if possible.

FURTHER READING

Gillon R (1986) The principle of double effect and medical ethics. BMJ (Clin Res Ed) 292(6514):193–194 (Free PDF Available Online via PubMed)

Hallenbeck J (2005) Palliative care in the final days of life: "they were expecting it at any time". JAMA 293(18):2265–2271

Hudson PL, Schofield P, Kelly B, Hudson R, O'Connor M, Kristjanson LJ, Ashby M, Aranda S (2006) Responding to desire to die statements from patients with advanced disease: recommendations for health professionals. Palliat Med 20(7):703–710

Sinclair CT, Stephenson R (2006) Palliative sedation: assessment, management, and ethics. Hosp Phys 42(3):33–42 (Free PDF Available Online via www.turner-white.com)

Storey CP, Levine S, Shega JW (2008) UNIPAC Series, 3rd edn, vol 1–9. AAHPM, Glenview, IL

Index

A
Acetaminophen, 33
Activities of daily living scale, 31
Acute depression, 22
Anorexia, 15
Anticipatory grief, 4–5
Anticipatory nausea, 47
Anticonvulsants, 22, 26
Antidepressants, 21–24
Antipsychotics, 21, 26
Artificial nutrition and hydration (ANH), 15
Aspiration pneumonitis/pneumonia, 16

B
Benzodiazepines, 21, 23, 25
Bereavement, 5–6
Bi-level positive airway pressure (Bi-PAP)
    device, 38, 39
Bone pain, 53
Bowel obstruction, 48
Braden scale, 66
Breast cancer, 64

C
Cachexia, 15–17
Chronic obstructive pulmonary disease
    (COPD), 73
    disease-directed interventions, 39
    dyspnea (*see* Dyspnea)
    goals of care directed treatment plan,
      38–39
    mood, 41
    opioids, 39–40
    secretions, end of life, 42
Communication issues
    bad news, 8–9
    goals of care, 9–10
    hospice, 10
    prognosis, 11
    team communication, 11–12

Congestive heart failure (CHF). *See also*
    Heart failure
    diabetes mellitus, 29
    diuretics, 32
    fatigue, 30
    weight gain, 32
Constipation. *See also* Opioids
    causes, 44
    diarrhea, 45–46
    medication, 49
    methylnaltrexone, 2
    physical exam, 44
    therapeutic interventions, 45

D
Delirium, 23. *See also* Terminal delirium
Dexamethasone, 59
Diarrhea, 45–46
Diuretics, 32, 33
Dyspnea, 73. *See also* Chronic obstructive
    pulmonary disease (COPD)
    anxiety and depression, 41
    Bi-PAP, 39
    distress, 38
    heart failure, 32–33
    methylphenidate, 41
    mood, 41
    opioids, 39–40
    palliative sedation, 78
    treatment options, 39

E
Early satiety, 15
End-of-life care, 3–4
    hastened death, 77–78
    respiratory suppression, 77
    symptom management
      assessment, 75
      comprehensive education, 75
      foundation, 74

Lightning Source UK Ltd.
Milton Keynes UK
175180UK00003B/1/P

9 781607 615897